The Quick Reference

Medical Psychiatry:
The Quick Reference

MARY ANN L.C. BARNOVITZ, M.D.
General Psychiatry Resident
Department of Psychiatry and Behavioral Sciences
University of California, Davis
Sacramento, California

PRIA JOGLEKAR, M.D.
Chief Resident
Department of Psychiatry and Behavioral Sciences
University of California, Davis
Sacramento, California

Wolters Kluwer | Lippincott Williams & Wilkins
Health
Philadelphia · Baltimore · New York · London
Buenos Aires · Hong Kong · Sydney · Tokyo

Acquisitions Editor: Charles Mitchell
Managing Editor: Sirkka Bertling
Associate Director of Marketing: Adam Glazer
Project Manager: Fran Gunning
Art Director: Risa Clow
Compositor: International Typesetting and Composition

© 2008 Lippincott Williams & Wilkins, a Wolters Kluwer business
530 Walnut Street
Philadelphia, PA 19106
LWW.com

All rights reserved. This book is protected by copyright. No part of this book may be reproduced in any form or by any means, including photocopying, or utilizing by any information storage and retrieval system without written permission from the copyright owner, except for brief quotations embodied in critical articles and reviews.

Printed in the USA

Library of Congress Cataloging-in-Publication Data
Barnovitz, Mary Ann L. C.
  Medical psychiatry : the quick reference / Mary Ann L.C. Barnovitz, Pria Joglekar.
    p. ; cm.
  Includes bibliographical references and index.
  ISBN-13: 978-0-7817-7209-9
  ISBN-10: 0-7817-7209-5
  1. Psychiatry—Handbooks, manuals, etc. 2. Primary care (Medicine)—Handbooks, manuals, etc. I. Joglekar, Pria. II. Title.
  [DNLM: 1. Mental Health Services—organization & administration—Handbooks. 2. Mental Disorders—complications—Handbooks. 3. Psychiatry—methods—Handbooks. WM 34 B262m 2007]
  RC456.B37 2007
  616.89—dc22
                                                    2007016392

Care has been taken to confirm the accuracy of the information presented and to describe generally accepted practices. However, the authors, editors, and publisher are not responsible for errors or omissions or for any consequences from application of the information in this book and make no warranty, expressed or implied, with respect to the currency, completeness, or accuracy of the contents of the publication. Application of this information in a particular situation remains the professional responsibility of the practitioner.

The authors, editors, and publisher have exerted every effort to ensure that drug selection and dosage set forth in this text are in accordance with current recommendations and practice at the time of publication. However, in view of ongoing research, changes in government regulations, and the constant flow of information relating to drug therapy and drug reactions, the reader is urged to check the package insert for each drug for any change in indications and dosage and for added warnings and precautions. This is particularly important when the recommended agent is a new or infrequently employed drug.

Some drugs and medical devices presented in this publication have Food and Drug Administration (FDA) clearance for limited use in restricted research settings. It is the responsibility of health care providers to ascertain the FDA status of each drug or device planned for use in their clinical practice.

The publishers have made every effort to trace copyright holders for borrowed material. If they have inadvertently overlooked any, they will be pleased to make the necessary arrangements at the first opportunity.

To purchase additional copies of this book, call our customer service department at (800) 639-3030 or fax orders to (301) 824-7390. International customers should call (301) 714-2324. Lippincott Williams & Wilkins customer service representatives are available from 8:30 am to 6:00 pm, EST, Monday through Friday, for telephone access. Visit Lippincott Williams & Wilkins on the Internet: http://www.lww.com.

10 9 8 7 6 5 4 3 2 1

*For my husband Michael and my daughter Maya,
the focus of all my love and energy.*
—MB

For Amitabh.
—PJ

PREFACE

Our book came about three years ago as the result of the encouragement of an attending forensic psychiatrist, Dr. Cameron Quanbeck, and our desire for a quick reference handbook that encompassed the expanding scope of psychiatric care. It is not intended to turn psychiatrists into general medical practitioners or serve as an all-inclusive guide to manage every medical condition presenting in psychiatric settings. This manual provides psychiatrists with a quick and practical resource to provide superior medical and psychiatrically integrated patient care. In so doing, psychiatrists will improve the patient's overall health, strengthen the physician–patient therapeutic alliance, and minimize exposure to potential litigation stemming from nonadherence to the ever-evolving standard of care.

We would like to acknowledge the following individuals who were instrumental in the completion of this publication. Dr. Robert McCarron and Dr. Richard Bermudes advised us early on in developing the conceptual framework of this book and provided support and encouragement when we doubted the sanity and feasibility of our project. Dr. Malia McCarthy and Dr. John O'Neal assisted us in securing a publisher. Dr. Robert Hales assisted in securing permissions to utilize American Psychiatry Publishing, Inc. materials. Charley Mitchell, executive editor at Lippincott Williams & Wilkins, believed in our project and coordinated the approval of our manual for publication. Our families, especially our husbands, supported and tolerated our weekend work retreats which turned into weeklong retreats to complete this book.

Finally, we're amazed that our friendship survived this grueling undertaking and managed to flourish despite the overwhelming stresses of ongoing life, including chief residency and the birth of a baby girl.

CONTENTS

Preface vii

SECTION I ▪ COMMON MEDICAL CALLS

Chapter 1
Abdominal Pain 3

Chapter 2
Anaphylaxis 5

Chapter 3
EKG Interpretation 7

Chapter 4
Cellulitis 10

Chapter 5
Chest Pain 12

Chapter 6
Constipation 18

Chapter 7
Diabetes Mellitus 21

Chapter 8
Dyspepsia 25

Chapter 9
Dyspnea/Shortness of Breath 29

Chapter 10
Electrolyte Disturbances 31

Chapter 11
Emergency Contraception 37

x   Contents

Chapter 12
Falls   38

Chapter 13
Fever   40

Chapter 14
Viral Hepatitis   42

Chapter 15
Human Bite   45

Chapter 16
Hypertension   46

Chapter 17
Thyroid Disorders   52

Chapter 18
Metabolic Syndrome   54

Chapter 19
Nausea and Vomiting   56

Chapter 20
Tuberculosis Screening   59

Chapter 21
Smoking Cessation Pharmacotherapy   61

Chapter 22
Urinanalysis   63

Chapter 23
Urinary Tract Infections   65

SECTION II ▪ EMERGENT NEUROLOGIC CONDITIONS

Chapter 24
Headache   69

Chapter 25
Intracranial Hemorrhage   71

Chapter 26
Multiple Sclerosis 73

Chapter 27
Seizure Disorder 75

Chapter 28
Stroke Localization 78

Chapter 29
Transient Ischemic Attack/Stroke 79

SECTION III ▪ NEUROPSYCHIATRY

Chapter 30
Delirium 83

Chapter 31
Dementia 88

Chapter 32
Huntington Disease 97

Chapter 33
Parkinson Disease 99

Chapter 34
Sleep Disorders 102

Chapter 35
Traumatic Brain Injury 107

Chapter 36
HIV/AIDS 111

SECTION IV ▪ PSYCHIATRY

Chapter 37
Violence 121

Chapter 38
Capacity 125

Chapter 39
Alcohol Intoxication and Withdrawal 127

Chapter 40

Benzodiazepine Withdrawal   132

Chapter 41

Psychotropic-Induced Movement Disorders   134

Chapter 42

Substances of Abuse   138

Chapter 43

Electroconvulsive Therapy   145

Chapter 44

Malingering   149

Chapter 45

Postpartum Disorders   152

Chapter 46

Psychotropic Management in Pregnancy   156

Chapter 47

Use of Psychotropics in Breastfeeding   161

Chapter 48

Drug Overdose   164

Chapter 49

Drug-Induced Neurological Syndromes   170

Chapter 50

Physical Health Monitoring for Psychotropic Medications   175

Chapter 51

Suicide Assessment and Management   191

Chapter 52

Herbals and Dietary Supplements   194

SECTION V ▪ APPENDICES

Appendix 1

Initial Psychiatric Evaluation   203

Appendix 2
Mental Status Exam 205

Appendix 3
Neurologic Exam 207

Appendix 4
Neuropsychological Testing 209

Index 211

Medical Psychiatry:
The Quick Reference

Section I

Common Medical Calls

Chapter 1

ABDOMINAL PAIN

Location	Differential Diagnosis
Left upper quadrant	Splenic disease Myocardial infarction Dissecting aortic aneurysm Pneumonia Pyelonephritis Nephrolithiasis Pancreatitis Hiatal hernia Peptic ulcer disease Mallory-Weiss tear
Epigastrium	Peptic ulcer disease Esophagitis Myocardial infarction Pericarditis Pneumonia Pancreatitis Cholecystitis Perforation/obstruction
Right upper quadrant	Hepatitis Hepatic tumor Cholelithiasis Cholecystitis Cholangitis Pyelonephritis Nephrolithiasis Pneumonia Pulmonary embolism/infarction
Periumbilical	Gastroenteritis Appendicitis Pancreatitis Intestinal ischemia/infarction Intestinal obstruction
Left lower quadrant	Diverticulitis Colon cancer Urinary tract infection Nephrolithiasis Pyelonephritis Irritable bowel syndrome Gynecologic causes (ectopic pregnancy, pelvic inflammatory disease, mittelschmerz, ovarian cyst, fibroids, endometriosis, tumor, torsion) Inguinal hernia Psoas abscess

(*Continued*)

Location	Differential Diagnosis
Hypogastrium	Ectopic pregnancy Ovarian torsion Pelvic inflammatory disease

Right lower quadrant	Same as for left lower quadrant plus
	    Appendicitis
	    Diverticulitis
	    Meckel's diverticulum
	    Intussusception

Management of Acute Abdomen

- In the presence of signs and symptoms of acute abdomen, immediate medical and/or surgical consultation is critical.
- Monitor vital signs, maintain NPO (nothing by mouth) and hydration status.
- Features indicating a high-risk situation include guarding, writhing, lack of bowel sounds, inability to pass flatus, hypotension along with pulsatile abdominal mass (ruptured abdominal aortic aneurysm).
- Initial studies may include complete blood count (CBC) with differential q4h, CHEM 7, Ca, Mg, PO4, hepatic function, amylase, lipase, urine pregnancy test.
- Other studies as indicated may include electrocardiogram (EKG), upright chest X-ray, upright or left lateral decubitus and supine abdominal film, CT scan, ultrasound.

Chapter 2

ANAPHYLAXIS

Clinical features	Cutaneous—pruritus, urticaria, angioedema.
	Gastrointestinal—abdominal cramping, diarrhea.
	Vascular—hypotension.
	Respiratory—respiratory distress due to laryngeal edema, laryngospasm, or bronchospasm.
Immediate treatment	Initiate code blue.
	Assess airway, breathing, and circulation.
	Administer epinephrine 0.3–0.5 mg (0.3–0.5 ml of a 1:1000 solution) IM or SC.
	Repeat injections at 10- to 20-min intervals if necessary. Injection in the anterolateral thigh may lead to more predictable and rapid absorption compared with sites in the arm.
	Airway maintenance is a priority and endotracheal intubation or tracheostomy may be necessary.
	Antihistamines such as diphenhydramine (25–50 mg p.o./IV/IM) and ranitidine (150 mg p.o. q12h or 50 mg IM/IV q6–8 h) may shorten the duration of the reaction and ameliorate the cutaneous manifestations and gastrointestinal and uterine smooth muscle spasms.
	Respiratory therapy, albuterol/ipratropium bromide (Atrovent) nebulizers.
	Volume expansion with IV fluids may be necessary if the patient remains hypotensive.
	Observation for a minimum of 6 h is indicated for mild reactions.
	Moderate to severe reactions warrant hospitalization and close observation for 24 h.
Prevention	Identify the offending antigen.
	Record the offending antigen and document anaphylactic reaction.
	Ensure the chart is prominently marked to avoid exposure to the offending antigen during subsequent visits.
	Counsel patient regarding avoidance of the offending antigen and immediate management of future anaphylactic reactions.
	Refer patient to medicine or allergy/immunology for further evaluation and long-term prophylactic treatment as indicated.
	Self-administered epinephrine may be prescribed for patients with a history of anaphylaxis.

References

Green GB, Harris IS, Lin GA, et al., eds. *The Washington Manual of Medical Therapeutics.* 31st ed. Philadelphia: Lippincott Williams & Wilkins; 2004: 233–234.

Tierney LM, McPhee SJ, Papadakis MA. *2006 Current Medical Diagnosis and Treatment.* 45th ed. New York: McGraw-Hill; 2006:791–792.

Chapter 3

EKG INTERPRETATION

1. Determine the **rate** = 300 divided by the number of large boxes between two successive QRS complexes.
   - Normal rate = 60–100 beats per minute.
   - Bradycardia <60
   - Tachycardia >100
2. Determine the **rhythm.** Is it regular, irregular, or irregularly irregular?
   - Normal sinus rhythm—
     - 60–100 beats per minute.
     - Each P wave followed by QRS.
     - P wave upright in leads I, II, III.
     - PR interval >0.12 sec (three small boxes).
   - With junctional rhythm, there is loss of P waves and rate is 40–60 beats per minute.
   - With ventricular rhythm the rate is 20–40 beats per minute.
3. Determine the **axis.**
   - QRS complex in leads I and aVF are positive indicates axis is normal.
   - QRS complex up in lead I and down in lead aVF indicates left axis deviation—think left anterior fascicular block, left ventricular hypertrophy, inferior wall myocardial infarction.
   - QRS complex down in lead I and up in lead aVF indicates right axis deviation—think right ventricular hypertrophy, acute right heart strain (e.g., massive pulmonary embolism), left posterior fascicular block.
4. Determine the **intervals.**
   - Normal PR = 0.12–0.20 sec (three to five small boxes).
   - Normal QRS = ≤0.10sec (≤2.5 small boxes).
   - QTc should be <440 msec (less than half of RR interval).
   - Corrected QT = QT interval divided by the square root of (RR interval).
5. **P wave abnormalities.**
   - In right atrial enlargement, the initial component of part of the P wave is prominent (>2.5 mm) in lead II.
   - In left atrial enlargement, there is a large terminal downward deflection in lead V1 and the terminal component of part of the P wave is prominent.
6. **QRS** wave abnormalities.
   - Inspect for Q waves, bundle branch blocks, and ventricular hypertrophy.
7. **Q waves.**
   - Significant Q waves are >25% of QRS height and duration >0.04 sec. Q waves indicate *necrosis* and may be due to old infarct. They remain for the lifetime of the patient.

8. Look at **R wave progression** across precordial leads.
   - Poor R wave progression may indicate an anterior infarction and is also seen with right ventricular hypertrophy, chronic obstructive pulmonary disease, and most commonly with improperly placed EKG leads.
9. **ST and T wave changes.**
   - ST segment changes indicate an acute process or *ongoing injury*.
   - ST elevations with significant Q waves indicate an acute or recent infarct.
   - ST depression that is persistent may represent subendocardial ischemia or infarct.
   - T wave inversion indicates *ongoing ischemia*.
   - Anatomical localization is determined by ST or T wave changes as follows:
     - II, III, aVF—inferior wall infarct with right coronary artery involvement.
     - V1, V2—anteroseptal infarct with left anterior descending artery involvement.
     - V3, V4—anteroapical infarct with left anterior descending artery distal involvement.
     - V5, V6, I, aVL—anterolateral infarct with circumflex involvement.
     - V1, V2 (tall R, not Q)—posterior infarct with right coronary artery involvement.
10. **Bundle branch blocks.**
    - RBBB—QRS in V1 is positive. Widened QRS (>0.12 sec), RSR' in leads V1 and V2 (rabbit ears), ST segment depression, T wave inversion.
    - LBBB—Widened QRS (>0.12 sec), broad or notched R wave with prolonged upstroke in leads V5, V6, I, aVL with ST segment depression and T wave inversion.
11. **Hypertrophy.**
    - Right ventricular hypertrophy—R > S in lead V1 and right axis deviation.
    - Left ventricular hypertrophy—S in V1 with R in V5 or V6 ≥ 35 mm or R in aVL >11 mm or R in lead I >15 mm.
12. **Arrythmias.**
    - Tachyarrhythmias (>100 beats per minute).
      - Narrow QRS complex rhythms (≤0.12 sec).
        - Regular rhythm—sinus tachycardia, supraventricular tachycardia (SVT), atrial flutter.
        - Irregular rhythm—atrial fibrillation, multifocal atrial tachycardia.
      - Wide QRS complex rhythms (>0.12 sec)
        - Monomorphic or polymorphic ventricular tachycardia, supraventricular tachycardia (SVT) with aberrant conduction, ventricular fibrillation.
    - Bradyarrhythmias (<60 beats per minute).
      - First-degree atrioventricular (AV) block—PR interval prolongation (>0.2 sec) and every P wave is followed by a QRS complex.

- Second-degree AV block—every P wave is not followed by a QRS complex in an intermittent manner.
    - Mobitz type I block (Wenckebach block)—progressive prolongation in the PR interval from one beat to the next until a single QRS complex is dropped.
    - Mobitz type II block—series of cycles consisting of one normal complete conduction cycle preceded by a series of paced P waves that fail to conduct through the AV node.
    - Third-degree AV block—P waves and QRS complexes occur independent of each other.
13. **Prolonged QTc interval.**
    - Causes include medications, electrolyte disturbances, hypothermia, myocardial infarction, intracranial hemorrhage, and congenital disorders.
    - Medication-induced causes include neuroleptic agents (thioridazine > ziprasidone > haloperidol, quetiapine, resperidone, olanzapine), tricyclics, high-dose methadone, droperidol, cocaine, antiarrhythmics (e.g., amiodarone, quinidine), antimicrobials, antihistamines (e.g., fexofenadine).
    - QTc prolongation can lead to the development of torsades de pointes which can result in sudden cardiac death. Risk factors for drug-induced torsades de pointes include female gender, baseline risk factors for arrhythmia (e.g., electrolyte disturbance, pre-existing arrhythmias, baseline prolonged QTc interval), bradycardia, digitalis therapy, pre-existing cardiac disease (e.g., heart failure).
14. Compare with patient's previous EKGs.

References

Dubin D. *Rapid Interpretation of EKG's*. 6th ed. Tampa: COVER Publishing Company; 2000.

Low K, Kerfoot P, Lilly LS. Electrocardiogram. In: Lilly LS, ed. *Pathophysiology of Heart Disease*. 2nd ed. Baltimore: Lippincott Williams & Wilkins; 1998:65–99.

Manu P, Suarez RE, Barnett BJ, eds. *Handbook of Medicine in Psychiatry*. Arlington: American Psychiatric Publishing, Inc; 2006:459–489.

Thaler, MS. *The Only EKG Book You'll Ever Need*. 3rd ed. Baltimore: Lippincott Williams & Wilkins; 1999.

Chapter 4

CELLULITIS

Pathogens	Gram-positive cocci, especially Beta-hemolytic *Streptococcus* **or** *Staphylococcus aureus*.
Clinical features	Most commonly on the lower extremities.
	Predisposing factors may include tinea pedis of the toe web with fissuring, IV drug use, open ulcerations, diabetes.
	Presence of *tenderness*, erythema, and edema.
	May be accompanied by systemic symptoms, such as chills, fever, and malaise progressing to septicemia.
	Blood studies show leukocytosis and neutrophilia, and blood cultures may be positive.
Differential diagnosis	Deep venous thrombosis.
	Necrotizing fasciitis.
	Acute severe contact dermatitis.
Management	Consult medicine to determine severity of cellulitis (particularly patients with moderate to severe disease, diabetes, and immunocompromised status) and guidance regarding further treatment.
	IV antibiotics may be required for the first 24–72 h.
	Possible cases warranting IV antibiotics include large area associated with systemic symptoms, deep ulcer, osteomyelitis, abscess, comorbid diabetes.
	Mild cases or following initial IV therapy, administer dicloxacillin or cephalexin 250–500 mg QID for 5–10 d.
	Additionally, demarcate the area of the cellulitis, elevate extremity, and apply warm compresses to infected area TID.
	Culture may be indicated in the presence of an ulcer, pustule, or abscess.
	If present, treat coexisting tinea pedis with topical antifungals to prevent recurrence of lower extremity cellulitis.
	Ensure diabetic patients receive counseling regarding periodic foot examination and the importance of foot hygiene and properly fitting shoe gear.

References

Green GB, Harris IS, Lin GA, et al., eds. *The Washington Manual of Medical Therapeutics*. 31st ed. Philadelphia: Lippincott Williams & Wilkins; 2004:295.

Tierney LM, McPhee SJ, Papadakis MA. *2006 Current Medical Diagnosis and Treatment*. 45th ed. New York: McGraw-Hill Companies, Inc; 2006:124–125.

Chapter 5

CHEST PAIN

General Considerations

- Chest pain may be the first sign of a medical emergency and needs immediate attention. Always evaluate in person and immediately.
- When called about a patient complaining of chest pain ask the following:
  - Severity, onset, nature, location, quality, and duration of the pain.
  - Vital signs.
  - History of cardiovascular disease (myocardial infarction [MI], angina, hypertension [HTN]) and if the pain is similar to past anginal episodes.
  - Age.
  - Admitting diagnosis, including toxicology screen results.
- Order a stat EKG and vital signs, including blood pressures in both arms.

Differential Diagnosis of Chest Pain

Cardiovascular	*Angina*
	Myocardial infarction
	Aortic dissection
	Myocarditis
	Pericarditis
	Valvular heart disease
Pulmonary	Pleuritis
	Pneumonia
	Pulmonary embolism
	Tension pneumothorax
Gastrointestinal	Biliary disease
	Esophageal spasm/reflux
	Esophageal rupture
	Pancreatitis
	Peptic ulcer disease, *perforating* vs non-perforating
	Mallory-Weiss tear
Musculoskeletal	Cervical disc disease
	Costochondritis
	Herpes zoster
	Neuropathic pain
	Rib fracture
	Muscle spasm/strain
Psychiatric	Anxiety
	Somatoform disorders
	Pain disorder
	Somatic delusions
	Factitious disorder
	Malingering
	Cocaine and/or amphetamine intoxication

Note: Italics indicate potentially life-threatening conditions.

Management and Differentiation of Various Causes of Chest Pain

Differential	Symptoms	Signs	Workup While Awaiting Transfer	Initial Managment
Myocardial ischemia *The earlier thrombolytic therapy is started, the better the outcome. Therefore, transfer to a cardiac care unit ASAP is critical.*	Radiates to the neck or arms, palpitations, diaphoresis, shortness of breath, nausea/vomiting.	EKG may reveal T wave inversion, ST elevation/depression and Q waves. Compare with an old EKG. Examine for heart failure, hypotension (ominous), new S4 or murmurs.	Vital signs, O_2 saturations Q15. CPK-MB and troponin stat, then serially by cardiac care team. CBC, CHEM 7, Ca, Mg, PO4.	Page medicine stat. and prepare to transfer patient. Aspirin (ASA) 325 mg chewed × 1 stat O_2 2 L by nasal cannula. Continuous cardiac monitoring. Ensure IV access and rule out hypotension before nitroglycerin (NTG) administration. NTG 0.4 mg SL q5min × 3 prn continued chest pain, hold for systolic BP <100. Consider beta-blocker therapy/ACE inhibitor therapy.
Aortic dissection	Tearing pain in the chest or upper back radiating to the neck and jaw, abdomen. Lacks squeezing quality or pressure of myocardial ischemia.	Diminished or unequal peripheral pulses and blood pressures. Syncope, hypotension. Neurologic deficits such as hemiplegia or lower extremity paralysis. EKG may be normal or reveal acute ischemic changes, left ventricular hypertrophy (LVH).	Vital signs, O_2 saturations q15min. Type and cross match blood for possible surgery and/or rupture. Immediate workup may entail stat thoracic and/or abdominal CT/MRI scanning or transesophageal echocardiogram.	Page medicine and surgery stat. and prepare to transfer patient. Emergent medical treatment entails beta-blockade followed by vasodilation. Control pain with MSO_4^{2-} Prn.

(Continued)

Management and Differentiation of Various Causes of Chest Pain (continued)

Differential	Symptoms	Signs	Workup While Awaiting Transfer	Initial Managment
Pericarditis *Pericardial tamponade, requiring urgent intervention, presents with distant heart sounds, jugular venous distension, and hypotension.*	Usually pleuritic pain (exacerbated by inhalation, coughing, sneezing), often relieved by sitting and/or leaning forward. Radiates to the back, neck, and/or shoulder. Fever.	Pericardial friction rub. Distant heart sounds if pericardial effusion present. EKG may reveal ST elevation, PR depression, T wave inversion.	Vital signs, O_2 saturations q15min. CBC, CHEM 7. Chest x-ray. Transthoracic echocardiogram. Further workup may entail pericardiocentesis or biopsy for microbiologic and cytologic studies, as well as evaluation for infectious and noninfectious etiologies.	Page medicine stat. Ibuprofen 800 mg PO q6h with food. Avoid anticoagulants. Further management as determined by etiology and medicine recommendations.
Pulmonary embolism (PE)	Pleuritic chest pain, shortness of breath, fever, hemoptysis.	Hypoxemia, pleural rub, new right-sided heart failure, and tachycardia. Signs and symptoms of deep venous thrombosis (DVT) increase risk of PE.	Vital signs, O_2 saturations q15min. CBC and coagulation studies. Chest x-ray. EKG. Arterial blood gases. D-dimer. Further workup may entail venous duplex scan, V/Q scan, spiral chest CT and/or pulmonary angiogram.	Page medicine stat. Further management as per medicine.

(Continued)

Management and Differentiation of Various Causes of Chest Pain (continued)

Differential	Symptoms	Signs	Workup While Awaiting Transfer	Initial Managment
Pneumothorax *Tension pneumothorax, requiring urgent intervention, presents with hypotension, respiratory distress, and history of mechanical ventilation and/or procedure involving piercing of the thorax.*	Usually abrupt onset of shortness of breath, pleuritic chest pain, cough.	Involved hemithorax may be larger and relatively immobile during respiration. Accessory muscle usage. Pursed lip breathing. On lung exam, decreased breath sounds, decreased vocal fremitus, more resonant percussion note.	Vital signs, O_2 saturations q15min. Arterial blood gases. Chest x-ray. EKG may be misinterpreted as acute myocardial infarction.	Page medicine stat. O_2 2 L by nasal cannula. Large, progressive, or tension pneumothorax may require emergent thoracentesis with subsequent chest tube placement.
Gastritis and peptic ulcer disease *Ulcer perforation, requiring urgent intervention, presents with "coffee ground" emesis, hematemesis, melena or hematochezia, epigastric pain, syncope.*	Epigastric pain described as burning, gnawing, "hunger-like." Anorexia, nausea, vomiting. History of NSAIDs, alcohol, severe stress, burn injuries.	Mild, localized epigastric tenderness to deep palpation may be present. Hematemesis, melena.	CBC. Guiaic stools ×3. Esophagogastroduodenoscopy. Testing for *Helicobacter pylori*.	Discontinue NSAIDs, smoking, heavy alcohol, caffeine. Further treatment with H_2 blockers/proton pump inhibitors/antacids as recommended. Potential pharmacotherapy may include famotidine 40 mg p.o. qhs, ranitidine 300 mg p.o. qhs, esomeprazole 40 mg p.o. QD, lansoprazole 30 mg po QD, pantoprazole 40 mg p.o. QD and/or *H. pylori* eradication treatment.

(Continued)

Management and Differentiation of Various Causes of Chest Pain (continued)

Differential	Symptoms	Signs	Workup While Awaiting Transfer	Initial Managment
Acute pancreatitis	Severe, constant, boring midepigastric or lower chest pain, radiating to the back. Nausea, vomiting. Fever.	Abdominal tenderness, distension, and guarding. Fever, tachycardia, hypotension. Mild jaundice. +/− palpable abdominal mass.	Amylase. Lipase. CBC. CHEM 7, Ca, Mg, PO4. Hepatic function. Further workup may include abdominal CT and/or abdominal-pelvic ultrasound, endoscopic retrograde cholangio-pancreatography (ERCP).	Page medicine and surgery stat. Keep NPO (nothing by mouth). Treatment necessitates inpatient admission and may involve fluid resuscitation, pain management, and electrolyte repletion.
Musculoskeletal	Usually reproducible. Common causes include costochondritis, cervical disc disease, osteoarthritis, rib fractures, herpes zoster.	Unremarkable vital signs, chest x-ray, EKG.	Vital signs. Chest x-ray. EKG.	NSAIDs.

References

Breen L, Barnett B. Chest pain. In: Manu P, Suarez RE, Barnett BJ, eds. *Handbook of Medicine in Psychiatry*. Arlington: American Psychiatric Publishing, Inc; 2006:97–104.

Green GB, Harris IS, Lin GA, et al., eds. *The Washington Manual of Medical Therapeutics*. 31st ed. Philadelphia: Lippincott Williams & Wilkins; 2004.

Rosen, H. *The Consult Manual of Internal Medicine*. Med Consult Publishing Inc; 2006.

Sabatine MS, ed. *The Massachusetts General Hospital Handbook of Internal Medicine*. Philadelphia: Lippincott Williams & Wilkins; 2000.

Tierney LM, McPhee SJ, Papadakis MA. *2006 Current Medical Diagnosis and Treatment*. 45th ed. New York: McGraw-Hill Companies, Inc; 2006.

Chapter 6

CONSTIPATION

Etiology	**Functional**
	Sedentary lifestyle or prolonged immobilization
	Low-fiber diet
	Low fluid intake
	Poor bowel habits, including ignoring the urge to defecate
	Pregnancy
	Medications
	Anticholinergics
	Antidepressants, particularly tricyclic antidepressants
	Antipsychotics, particularly clozapine and olanzapine
	Calcium channel blockers
	Cholestyramine
	Clonidine
	Diuretics
	Narcotics
	Calcium
	Iron
	Sucralfate
	Nonsteroidal anti-inflammatory drugs
	Opiates
	Systemic disease
	Hypothyroidism
	Diabetes
	Hypercalcemia
	Multiple sclerosis
	Paraplegia
	Uremia
	Motility disturbance
	Slow transit time
	Outlet delay
	Irritable bowel syndrome
	Structural abnormalities, including pain due to defecation and obstruction
	Anal stricture or fissure
	Colonic mass/stricture
	Hemorrhoids
	Psychogenic conditions
	Anxiety
	Depression
	Eating disorders
	Somatization

Pharmacologic Management of Constipation
Initial Management

- History and physical examination, including digital rectal exam and stool testing for occult blood.
- In order to rule out fecal impaction and obstruction, ask about abdominal bloating and cramping, recent weight loss, absence of flatus, and rectal bleeding.
- Labs may include CBC, CHEM 7, Ca, thyroid-stimulating hormone (TSH).
- Immediate radiologic studies may include abdominal x-ray to rule out obstruction.
- Presence of anemia, occult blood in stools, advanced age, recent change in bowel habits, acute onset of constipation, and those not responsive to conservative treatment require medical consultation.
- Bowel hygiene
  - Ensure adequate fluid intake, proper fiber intake, and regular exercise.
- Before initiating pharmacotherapy, ensure fecal impaction/obstruction/acute abdomen has been addressed.
- Enemas may be indicated for fecal impaction. Consider surgical consult at this point. Common agents include tap water, soapsuds, mineral oil, phosphate, and sulfates.

Commonly Used Agents	Dosing	Special Considerations
Fiber supplementation		Increase fluid intake. Gas and flatulence can occur, though less so with methylcellulose. Transient distention common.
Dietary fiber intake	Increase to 20–30 g/d	
Psyllium (Metamucil)	1 tsp QD-BID	
Methylcellulose (Citrucel)	1 tsp QD-BID	
Stool surfactants		
Docusate sodium (Colace)	100 mg p.o. QHS-BID	Increase fluid intake.
Osmotic laxatives		
Magnesium hydroxide (MOM)	15–30 ml p.o. QD-BID	Avoid in renal failure and cardiac disease due to risk of electrolyte imbalance.
Lactulose	15–30 ml p.o. BID-TID	Lactulose can cause cramps, bloating, and flatulence.
Stimulant laxatives	10–15 mg p.o. QHS or 10 mg PR prn	Avoid daily and chronic use.
Bisacodyl (Dulcolax)		
Senna	8.6–17.2 mg p.o. QD-TID	May cause cramps.
Prokinetic agent	6 mg p.o. BID	May benefit women with constipation-predominant irritable bowel syndrome.
Tegaserod (Zelnorm)		

References

Green GB, Harris IS, Lin GA, et al., eds. *The Washington Manual of Medical Therapeutics.* 31st ed. Philadelphia: Lippincott Williams & Wilkins; 2004:295.

Manu P, Suarez RE, Barnett BJ, eds. *Handbook of Medicine in Psychiatry.* Arlington: American Psychiatric Publishing, Inc; 2006:239–245.

Tierney LM, McPhee SJ, Papadakis MA. *2006 Current Medical Diagnosis and Treatment.* 45th ed. New York: McGraw-Hill Companies, Inc; 2006:124–125.

Chapter 7

DIABETES MELLITUS

General Considerations
- Normal glucose tolerance is defined by fasting plasma glucose <100 mg/dL.
- Impaired fasting glucose is defined by fasting plasma glucose 100–125 mg/dL.
- Impaired glucose tolerance and impaired fasting glucose are associated with insulin resistance and appear to be risk factors for type 2 diabetes mellitus and micro/macrovascular complications.

Diagnostic Criteria for Diabetes Mellitus
- Fasting plasma glucose ≥126 mg/dL with confirmatory repeat test.
- Random plasma glucose ≥200 mg/dL in the presence of symptoms, including polyuria, polydipsia, weakness, recurrent blurred vision, vulvovaginitis or pruritus, peripheral neuropathy.
- 2-h oral glucose tolerance test ≥200 mg/dL.

General Management Principles
- Coordinate care with primary care provider for management of diabetes mellitus, including monitoring for secondary complications and treatment of metabolic syndrome when present.
- Individuals with schizophrenia appear to have increased risk for diabetes mellitus, possibly due to a direct genetic link, but also secondary to weight gain, poor dietary habits, sedentary lifestyle, poor health habits (e.g., smoking) and treatment with atypical antipsychotics (particularly, clozapine and olanzapine).
- Additionally, other psychiatric medications (e.g., mood stabilizers, antidepressants) associated with weight gain may secondarily increase risk for diabetes mellitus.
- Dietary modification, including referral to a nutrition specialist.
- Regular exercise, weight loss.
- Smoking cessation.
- Self-monitoring of blood glucose.

Oral Antidiabetic Agents

Agent	Recommended Starting Dose (mg/day)	Dose(s) per of Day	Special Mechanism Action	Considerations/Precautions
Sulfonylureas			Stimulate pancreatic beta islet cell insulin secretion. Increased extra-pancreatic receptor sensitivity and number.	Hypoglycemia, weight gain.
Glyburide (Micronase, DiaBeta) (Glynase)	1.25–2.5 (max 20) 1.5–3 (max 12)	1–2 1–2		
Glipizide (Glucotrol) (Glucotrol XL)	2.5–5 (max 20) 2.5–5 (max 20)	1–2 1		
Glimepiride (Amaryl)	1–2 (max 8)	1		
Biguanides			Decrease hepatic gluconeogenesis. Increase insulin sensitivity.	Contraindicated in cardiac, renal, and/or liver failure, particularly with history of alcoholism. Gastrointestinal (GI) intolerance, lactic acidosis. Weight loss.
Metformin HCl (Glucophage)	500 (max 2000)	2–3		
Metformin HCL ER (Fortamet, Glucophage)	500 (max 2000)	1–2		
Alpha-glucosidase inhibitors			Decrease complex carbohydrate digestion by inhibiting alpha-glucosidase. Delay gastrointestinal absorption of carbohydrates.	GI intolerance, flatulence, abdominal discomfort, diarrhea greatest upon initiation of treatment; therefore, slow titration recommended.
Acarbose (Precose)	25 (max 300)	3		
Miglitol (Glyset)	25 (max 300)	3		
Thiazolidinediones			Decrease hepatic gluconeogenesis. Increase glucose uptake in muscle and adipose tissue. Decrease fatty acid release from adipose tissue. Increase insulin sensitivity.	Fluid retention, heart failure, hepatotoxicity, weight gain. Perform baseline hepatic function before initiating treatment; coordinate further hepatic monitoring with primary care provider.
Rosiglitazone (Avandia)	2 (max 8)	1–2		
Pioglitazone (Actos)	15 (max 45)	1		
Meglitinides			Increase pancreatic islet beta cell insulin secretion with faster onset and shorter duration compared to sulfonylureas.	Hypoglycemia, weight gain.
Repaglinide (Prandin)	0.5–1 (max 24)	2–4		
Nateglinide (Starlix)	60–120 (max 360)	2–4		

Oral Antidiabetic Agents Plus Insulin Therapy

- Patients with fasting plasma glucose <200 mg/dL, with symptoms, type 1 diabetes mellitus, underweight, and/or ketotic require insulin therapy. Determine agent and dosage regimen after consulting with medicine.
- Sliding scale for insulin adjustment is used to compensate for failure of glycemic control by the existing antidiabetic regimen. If the sliding scale is repetitively used, the existing antidiabetic regimen likely requires adjustment.

Sliding Scale for Insulin Adjustment

Blood Glucose (mg/dL)	Units of Regular Insulin Given
<60	1 ampule D50 or orange juice Call MD. Consider subtraction of 4 units from bedtime dose
60–150	No insulin
151–200	2 units
201–250	4 units
251–300	6 units
301–350	8 units and plenty of fluids
351–400	10 units
>400	12 units and call MD.

Distinguishing Features of Diabetic Ketoacidosis and Hyperglycemic Hyperosmolar State

Features	Diabetic Ketoacidosis (DKA)	Hyperglycemic Hyperosmolar State (HHS)
Precipitating factors	Infection, myocardial ischemia, trauma, surgery, insulin deficiency, alcohol and drug abuse.	Dehydration, noncompliance with medications, dietary indiscretion, impaired glucose excretion in patients with compromised renal function, plus precipitating factors for DKA.
Clinical features	Type 1 > Type 2 Nausea, vomiting. Dehydration. Vaguely localized abdominal pain. Deep and rapid respirations with a fruity odor (acetone). Hypotension. Altered mental status, obtundation, coma.	Type 2 > Type 1 Dehydration including tachycardia, hypotension, dry mucous membranes, decreased skin turgor. Lethargy and confusion, progressing to convulsions and deep coma.

(Continued)

Features	Diabetic Ketoacidosis (DKA)	Hyperglycemic Hyperosmolar State (HHS)
Diagnostic studies	Blood glucose >250 mg/dL. Anion gap (anion gap = Na −(Cl + HCO3)). Normal anion gap = 8–12 mEq/L. Metabolic acidosis with blood pH <7.3. Serum bicarbonate <15 mEq/L. Serum and urine ketones.	Blood glucose >600 mg/dL. Normal anion gap. No acidosis with blood pH >7.3. Serum bicarbonate >15 mEq/L. Ketosis absent or mild. Serum osmolality >310 mosm/kg.
Management	Consult medicine immediately. DKA is a medical emergency and ideally should be managed in an intensive care setting. Management involves aggressive hydration, insulin replacement, electrolyte repletion, and evaluation and treatment of underlying cause.	Consult medicine immediately. HHS is a medical emergency and ideally should be managed in an intensive care setting. Mortality rate is ten times that of DKA due to the higher incidence in older patients, severe dehydration, and delays in recognition and treatment. Management involves aggressive hydration, insulin replacement, electrolyte repletion, and evaluation and treatment of underlying cause.

References

Ahmadian M, Duckworth WC. Practical medical management of type 2 diabetes mellitus. *Resid. Staff Physician.* 2004;50(12):28–32.

Emerson P, Felicetta JV. Emerging treatments for diabetes mellitus type 1 or type 2: recently approved medications and more in the pipeline. *Resid. Staff Physician.* 2006;52(3):7–11.

Green GB, Harris IS, Lin GA, et al., eds. *The Washington Manual of Medical Therapeutics.* 31st ed. Philadelphia: Lippincott Williams & Wilkins; 2004:475–482, 479.

Manu P, Suarez RE, Barnett BJ, eds. *Handbook of Medicine in Psychiatry.* Arlington: American Psychiatric Publishing, Inc; 2006:419–428.

Rosen, H. *The Consult Manual of Internal Medicine.* Med Consult Publishing Inc; 2006:361–385.

Sabatine MS, ed. *The Massachusetts General Hospital Handbook of Internal Medicine.* Philadelphia: Lippincott Williams & Wilkins; 2000:7-12–7-14.

Tierney LM, McPhee SJ, Papadakis MA. *2006 Current Medical Diagnosis and Treatment.* 45th ed. New York: McGraw-Hill Companies, Inc; 2006:1213, 1227–1232.

Chapter 8

DYSPEPSIA

General Considerations

- Dyspepsia—pain or discomfort centered in the upper abdomen.
- Etiologies include food and/or drug intolerance, peptic ulcer disease, gastroesophageal reflux disease, *Helicobacter pylori*-associated gastritis, pancreatic disease, biliary tract disease, intraabdominal malignancy, pregnancy, myocardial infarction, and renal insufficiency.
- Dyspepsia is commonly present in psychiatric populations, largely due to the higher prevalence of comorbid alcohol and drug use and anticholinergic effects of psychiatric medications.

Management of Common Causes of Dyspepsia

Syndrome	Clinical Features	Diagnosis	Treatment
Gastroesophageal reflux disease (GERD)	"Heartburn"—substernal chest discomfort/pain with a burning quality. Difficulty swallowing and/or pain on swallowing (if associated with esophagitis). "Water brash"—sour or bitter taste in the mouth. Nocturnal cough (due to aspiration), asthma exacerbation, hoarseness of voice (due to vocal cord involvement). Increased risk of aspiration pneumonia. Precipitated by alcohol, caffeine, medications (such as anticholinergics, benzodiazepines), cigarette smoking, large meals, caffeine, fatty foods, and supine position.	Often a clinical diagnosis. 24-h pH monitoring. In the presence of dysphagia, odynophagia, early satiety, weight loss, or bleeding, and atypical symptoms (e.g., cough, asthma, hoarseness, chest pain), refer early for endoscopic evaluation.	Conservative measures: Smoking and alcohol cessation. Elevate head of bed at least 6 in. Small, frequent meals while avoiding late meals. Avoidance of medications and substances that may cause precipitation of symptoms (e.g. caffeine, fatty and spicy foods). Medications: After failure of lifestyle changes for 3 weeks and with complicated cases. H_2 blockers: May require long-term maintenance with half of acute treatment doses. Acute treatment doses are as follows: Famotidine (Pepcid) 40 mg p.o. at bedtime or 20 mg p.o. twice daily. Ranitidine (Zantac) 300 mg p.o. at bedtime or 150 mg p.o. twice daily. Side effects—Altered mental status, depression, constipation, diarrhea, headache, and thrombocytopenia in elderly patients. Caution with using cimetidine in psychiatric populations as it can cause delirium, and increase blood levels of valproic acid, selective serotonin reuptake inhibitors, carbamazepine, and tricyclics. Symptoms persisting despite a 6-week trial of acute treatment doses with H_2 blockers require treatment with proton pump inhibitors. Proton pump inhibitors: May require long-term maintenance with full acute treatment doses daily. Acute treatment doses are as follows:

(Continued)

Syndrome	Clinical Features	Diagnosis	Treatment
			Omeprazole (Prilosec) 40 mg p.o. daily. Has been reported to lower serum levels of clozapine. Lansoprazole (Prevacid) 30 mg p.o. daily. Pantoprazole (Protonix) 40 mg p.o. daily. Side effects—gastrointestinal upset, headaches, vitamin B_{12} deficiency with chronic use. For complicated and/or refractory cases refer to medicine/gastroenterology.
Peptic ulcer disease (PUD)	Can be asymptomatic. Epigastric abdominal pain (e.g., burning, tightness). Anorexia (especially with gastric involvement). Pain relieved by food (duodenal) and worsened by food (gastric). Nausea and vomiting. Upper GI bleed. Precipitated by NSAIDs, stress-related mucosal disease, alcohol, *H. pylori* infection.	*Helicobacter pylori* is causative agent for majority of ulcers. Testing for *H. pylori* may entail urea breath test, serology, EGD[a] + rapid urease, biopsy and histology. EGD is indicated if gastrointestinal tract (GI) bleed and/or neoplasia is suspected.	Conservative measures: Smoking and alcohol cessation. Discontinuation of NSAIDs including aspirin. Avoidance of precipitating dietary substances, including spicy food. Stress management techniques. Medications: *H. pylori*-associated PUD—treat with anti-*H. pylori* regimen ×10–14 d followed by maintenance with proton pump inhibitor/H_2 blocker ×4–8 weeks. Non-ulcer dyspepsia—trial of proton pump inhibitor. Acid suppressive treatment—maintenance treatment with proton pump inhibitor/H_2 blocker ×4–8 weeks, with continued treatment for complicated cases. Continue maintenance with H_2 blockers at half of acute treatment doses or proton pump inhibitors at full acute treatment doses. Refer to medicine for management in the event of evidence of GI bleed, perforation.

[a]EGD, esophagogastroduodenoscopy.

References

Manu P, Suarez RE, Barnett BJ, eds. *Handbook of Medicine in Psychiatry.* Arlington: American Psychiatric Publishing, Inc; 2006: 217–222.

Rosen, H. *The Consult Manual of Internal Medicine.* Med Consult Publishing Inc; 2006: 279–292.

Sabatine MS, ed. *The Massachusetts General Hospital Handbook of Internal Medicine.* Philadelphia: Lippincott Williams & Wilkins; 2000:3–2, 3–3, 3–4.

Tierney LM, McPhee SJ, Papadakis MA. *2006 Current Medical Diagnosis and Treatment.* 45th ed. New York: McGraw-Hill Companies, Inc; 2006: 586–591.

Chapter 9

DYSPNEA/SHORTNESS OF BREATH

Differential Diagnosis of Dyspnea

Cardiovascular	Congestive cardiac failure
	Acute myocardial infarction
	Cardiomyopathy
	Pericarditis
Pulmonary	Upper airway obstruction
	Asthma
	Chronic obstructive pulmonary disease
	Pleuritis
	Pneumonia
	Pulmonary embolism
	Pneumothorax
	Pleural effusion
	Acute respiratory distress syndrome
	Pulmonary fibrosis
Neurologic	Neuromuscular illness due to paralysis of respiratory muscles (e.g., myasthenia gravis, end-stage amyotrophic lateral sclerosis)
Metabolic	Metabolic acidosis
	Obesity-hypoventilation syndrome
Psychiatric	Dystonia
	Panic disorder
	Psychogenic dyspnea[a]

[a]Typically female patients between 20 and 40 years old, with attacks at rest and usually produced by stressful situations.

Assessment

- Do a preliminary examination, including checking the upper airways for any critical obstruction, respiratory rate, degree of obtundation and circulation (ABCs).
- Vital signs, including O_2 saturation.
- Bad prognostic factors:
  - Severe/worsening hypoxemia (with O_2 saturation <86%).
  - Change in mental status (lethargy, altered mental status, and coma).
  - Presence of symptoms and signs of acute coronary syndrome and pulmonary embolism.
- Page medicine/anesthesia stat if these are present.

- Check vitals, including O_2 saturation:
  - RR <12: consider stroke or narcotic overdose.
  - RR >24: consider hypoxia, pain, and anxiety.
- Heart and lung examination to check for wheezes, rhonchi, crackles and jugular venous distension, S3, and air movement.
  - Stridor—indicates upper airway obstruction and a need for intubation.
  - Wheezing—asthma, chronic obstructive pulmonary disease.
  - Diffuse basilar crackles—congestive heart failure, pulmonary fibrosis. Check for other signs suggestive of congestive cardiac failure, including peripheral edema, heart murmur.
  - Dullness on percussion—pleural effusion.
  - Unilateral absent breath sounds with increased tactile vocal fremitus—pneumothorax.
  - Hypotension—indicates possible congestive heart failure, pneumothorax, tension pnemothorax, and sepsis.
  - Unilateral leg edema—deep venous thrombosis, rule out pulmonary embolism.
- Assess mental status changes.

Management

- If psychiatric causes are thought to be unlikely, transfer to the medicine unit.
- Consider ordering the following studies while awaiting transfer:
  - Arterial blood gases.
  - EKG.
  - Stat. portable chest x-ray.
- Start O_2 by nasal cannula to keep O_2 saturation above 90%.
- Albuterol and Atrovent nebulizer if patient is wheezing.

References

Manu P, Suarez RE, Barnett BJ, eds. *Handbook of Medicine in Psychiatry.* Arlington: American Psychiatric Publishing, Inc; 2006:65–74.

Rosen, H. *The Consult Manual of Internal Medicine.* Med Consult Publishing Inc; 2006:202–212.

Chapter 10

ELECTROLYTE DISTURBANCES

Electrolyte	Etiology	Clinical Features	Management

Hypernatremia	Hypovolemic
	  Renal
	    Nephrogenic diabetes insipidus
	    Renal tubular dysfuntion
	    Medications (e.g., thiazide, loop diuretics)
	    Osmotic diuresis, including diabetic ketoacidosis, hyperosmolar hyperglycemic state
	  Nonrenal
	    Gastrointestinal (GI) fluid loss
	    Cutaneous fluid loss (e.g., severe burns, fever, heat exposure, mechanical ventilation)
	  Impaired thirst
	    Altered mental status, physically impaired, limited access to water
	Euvolemic
	  Diabetes insipidus (neurogenic or nephrogenic)
	Hypervolemic
	  Exogenous sodium infusion
		General
		  Anorexia
		  Fatigue
		  Irritability
		  Malaise
		  Restlessness
		  Fever
		  Flushed skin
		Neurologic
		  Delirium
		  Seizures
		  Coma
		  Hyperreflexia
		  Cerebral hemorrhage
		  Central pontine myelinolysis presenting with altered mental status, seizures, death
		Respiratory
		  Hyperventilation
		Gastrointestinal
		  Nausea/vomiting
			Consult medicine for plasma [Na^+] >145 mEq/L and presence of neurologic symptoms, mental status changes, hemodynamic instability, acute deterioration of renal function.
			Perform complete history and physical examination.
			Assess volume status, including vital signs, orthostatics, jugular venous distension, skin turgor, mucous membranes, edema.
			Confirm why patient is not drinking water (e.g., paranoia, catatonia, impaired mobility).
			Perform strict fluid intake/output measurements.
			Laboratory studies may entail chemistry panel, uric acid, urinalysis, urine Na/K/Cl, urine and serum osmolalities.
			Management as per medicine recommendations.
			Management of *lithium-induced nephrogenic diabetes insipidus*

(*Continued*)

Electrolyte	Etiology	Clinical Features	Management
	Hyperaldosteronism Hypercortisolism		(often reversible if lithium discontinued). Increase fluid intake. Consider K 10–20 mEq/day. Consider thiazide (caution), amiloride (nonthiazide and preferred) 5–10 mg p.o. BID. Discontinue lithium. Continue electrolyte monitoring. If lithium must be continued: Decrease to lowest effective dose and QD if able. Monitor lithium level minimum q2mos.
Hyponatremia	Hypotonic Hypovolemic Renal losses (e.g., diuretics, hypoaldosteronism) Extrarenal losses including GI, cutaneous. Euvolemic Syndrome of inappropriate antidiuretic hormone (most common cause) Medications (e.g., antipsychotics, antidepressants, thiazides) Hypothyroidism Adrenal insufficiency Primary polydipsia Psychogenic polydipsia Hypervolemic	General Anorexia Fatigue Malaise Agitation Hypothermia Orthostatic hypotension Neurologic Altered mental status Pseudobulbar palsy Cranial nerve palsies Hyporeflexia Positive Babinski sign Stupor Coma Seizures Death Lethargy	Consult medicine for plasma [Na$^+$] <130 mEq/L and/or rapid decrease in [Na$^+$] as well as presence of neurologic symptoms, mental status changes, hemodynamic instability, acute deterioration of renal function. Restrict fluid and perform close fluid intake/output measurements. Consider 1:1 observation if psychogenic polydipsia suspected. Perform complete history and physical examination. Assess volume status, including vital signs,

(*Continued*)

Electrolyte	Etiology	Clinical Features	Management

	Cirrhosis
	Congestive heart failure
	Nephrotic syndrome
	Advanced renal failure
	Isotonic
	  Pseudo-hyponatremia
	  Isotonic mannitol infusion
	Hypertonic
	  Hyperglycemia
	  Hypertonic solution infusions
		Respiratory Cheyne-Stokes respiration
		Gastrointestinal Ileus
		Nausea/vomiting
		Hiccups
		Musculoskeletal muscle cramps
			orthostatics, jugular venous distension, skin turgor, mucous membranes, edema.
			Laboratory studies may entail chemistry panel, uric acid, urinalysis, urine Na/K/Cl, urine and serum osmolalities.
			Management as per medicine recommendations.
			Generally, this involves determination and correction of etiology, cautious replacement of sodium and potassium, and fluid restriction/loss.
			Psychotropic-induced syndrome of inappropriate antidiuretic hormone secretion (SIADH):
			Antidepressants (selective serotonin reuptake inhibitors [SSRIs], tricyclic antidepressants [TCAs], venlafaxine), antipsychotics, and carbamazepine have been observed to cause SIADH.
			Symptoms include lethargy, headache, hyponatremia, elevated urinary sodium excretion, and hyperosmolar urine.
			Acute treatment generally involves discontinuation

(Continued)

Electrolyte	Etiology	Clinical Features	Management
			of drug and fluid restriction. If central nervous system (CNS) symptoms are present, refer to medicine for rapid correction of [Na$^+$]. Patients not responding to water restriction and discontinuation of drug may require demeclocycline therapy.
Hyperkalemia	Pseudohyperkalemia Hemolysis Marked leukocytosis Repeated fist clenching Transcellular shift Massive trauma, burns, neuromuscular disease Rhabdomyolysis Compartment syndrome (e.g., IV drug use) Massive blood transfusion Tumorlysis syndrome Metabolic acidosis Insulin deficiency Hypertonicity Exercise Beta-blockers Decreased K$^+$ excretion Renal failure Renal tubular dysfunction Hypoaldosteronism Medications including K$^+$ sparing diuretics, trimethoprim,	General Weakness Cardiovascular Bradycardia Peaked T waves (K$^+$ ≥5.5 mEq/L) AV conduction delay (K$^+$ ≥6.0 mEq/L) PR prolongation (K$^+$ >6.5 mEq/L) Widened QRS (K$^+$ ≥7.0 mEq/L) Dysrhythmias Gastrointestinal Nausea/ vomiting Abdominal distention Diarrhea Musculoskeletal Muscle weakness Rarely, flaccid paralysis, including	Stat. EKG. Consult medicine immediately in the event of severe hyperkalemia ([K$^+$] ≥6.0 mEq/L), EKG changes, and/or cardiac toxicity, muscular paralysis (even in the absence of EKG changes). Perform complete history (including medications and diet) and physical examination. In the absence of EKG changes and symptoms, recheck serum K level to rule out pseudohyperkalemia. Check chemistry panel, serum Ca, urine electrolytes, urine and serum osmolarities, creatine phosphokinase (CPK) level, urinalysis, urine toxicology screen, blood alcohol level. Mild hyperkalemia ([K$^+$] 5.0–5.5 mEq/L). Consider Kayexalate 30–60 g p.o./pr q6h prn. Repeat if no

(*Continued*)

Electrolyte	Etiology	Clinical Features	Management
	pentamidine, heparin, NSAIDs Diabetic nephropathy Excessive K^+ intake Iatrogenic	respiratory muscles Neurologic Hyporeflexia Paresthesias	bowel movement. Decreases $[K^+]$ by 0.5–1 mEq/L per dose.
Hypokalemia	Decreased K^+ intake Dietary restriction Transcellular shift Metabolic alkalosis Osmotic diuresis (e.g., hyperglycemia) Medications (e.g., beta-adrenergic agonists, insulin, barium) Anabolic states (e.g., rapidly proliferating malignancy) Hypothermia Hypokalemic periodic paralysis Renal loss Diuretic use/abuse Primary and secondary hyperaldosteronism Iatrogenic (e.g., loop and thiazide diuretics, antimicrobials, digoxin, licorice, tobacco, toluene, amphotericin B) Hypomagnesemia Renal tubular acidosis Cushing syndrome Diabetic	General Fatigue Cardiovascular AV conduction delay T wave flattening and/or inversion Prominent U wave ST depression Prolonged PR and QT interval Prolonged QU interval Gastrointestinal Nausea/vomiting Constipation/diarrhea Ileus Musculoskeletal Myalgia Muscular weakness/cramps, particularly of lower extremities Neurologic Hyporeflexia Paresthesias	Consult medicine for plasma $[K^+]$ <3mEq/L and presence of EKG changes, significant K^+ loss not responding to oral therapy and/or unable to tolerate oral therapy, patients taking digoxin. Perform complete history (including medications, past medical history, conditions predisposing to hypokalemia, such as bulimia and laxative abuse) and physical examination. Laboratory studies may entail chemistry panel, serum Mg and Ca, urine Na/K/Cl. Mild hypokalemia ($[K^+]$ 3.3–3.5 mEq/L) KCl 40–60 mEq/L p.o. in divided doses q2h. Moderate hypokalemia ($[K^+]$ 3.0–3.2 mEq/L) KCl 60–80 mEq/L p.o. in divided doses q2h.

(*Continued*)

Electrolyte	Etiology	Clinical Features	Management

	ketoacidosis
	Vomiting
	Nonrenal loss
	  Gastrointestinal loss (e.g., diarrhea, laxative, vomiting, nasogastric suction, Zollinger–Ellison syndrome, villous adenoma)
	  Excess sweating
	Pseudohyperkalemia
	  Lab error
	  Leukocytosis
			Continue monitoring serum K and serial EKGs until target serum $[K^+]$ 4–5 mEq/L.
			Replace serum Mg as needed.

References

Green GB, Harris IS, Lin GA, et al., eds. *The Washington Manual of Medical Therapeutics.* 31st ed. Philadelphia: Lippincott Williams & Wilkins; 2004:40–56.

Manu P, Suarez RE, Barnett BJ, eds. *Handbook of Medicine in Psychiatry.* Arlington: American Psychiatric Publishing, Inc; 2006:375–403.

Rosen, H. *The Consult Manual of Internal Medicine.* Med Consult Publishing Inc; 2006:850–865.

Sabatine MS, ed. *The Massachusetts General Hospital Handbook of Internal Medicine.* Philadelphia: Lippincott Williams & Wilkins; 2000:4-7 to 4-11.

Tierney LM, McPhee SJ, Papadakis MA. *2006 Current Medical Diagnosis and Treatment.* 45th ed. New York: McGraw-Hill Companies, Inc; 2006:866–876.

Chapter 11

EMERGENCY CONTRACEPTION

General Considerations

- Medicolegal considerations include ensuring adequate and detailed informed consent, presence of capacity to make medical decisions, and multidisciplinary management of victims recently sexually assaulted.
- Review applicable state guidelines prior to administration to an underage patient.
- Confirm patient is not currently pregnant.
- May be possible to administer emergency contraception within 120 h after unprotected sexual intercourse, but ideally as soon as possible.
- Adverse effects may include nausea and vomiting.
- An emergency contraception alternative may be IUD insertion within 5 d after one episode of unprotected midcyle intercourse.

Regimen	Frequency	Special Considerations
Lesvonorgestrel (0.75 mg). Also available as Plan B [2 pill sequential dosing packet labeled by the Food and Drug Administration (FDA)] for emergency contraception use).	Two doses 12 h apart.	1% failure rate when administered within 72 h of unprotected intercourse.
Ethinyl estradiol 50 mcg with norgestrel 0.5 mg. Also available as Preven.	Two tablets initially followed by two tablets 12 h later.	Ideally administer within 72 h of unprotected intercourse.

References

Tierney LM, McPhee SJ, Papadakis MA. *2006 Current Medical Diagnosis and Treatment.* 45th ed. New York: McGraw-Hill Companies, Inc; 2006:757.

Chapter 12

FALLS

Potential causes	Acute medical

Potential causes

Acute medical
- Myocardial infarction
- Arrhythmias
- Stroke
- Seizures
- Hypotension (rule out gastrointestinal bleed, sepsis, dehydration, drug-induced orthostasis, myocardial infarction)

Chronic medical
- Electrolyte abnormalities
- Metabolic disorders
- Vasovagal attacks

Psychiatric
- Delirium (particularly in patients taking narcotics, sedatives, tricyclic antidepressants, tranquilizers, cimetidine, and antihypertensives)
- Psychotropic-induced orthostatic hypotension and/or sedation (trazodone, quetiapine, chlorpromazine, tricyclic antidepressants)
- Dementia
- Purposeful fall, whether conscious or unconscious (such as psychotic, manic, patients with personality disorders, and somatoform disorders)
- Nonepileptiform seizures

Other
- Mechanical (patient disabled or ataxic)
- Visually impaired
- Multiple sensory deficits
- Environmental causes, including sun downing, wet floor, unassisted falls out of bed, walking without assistance

Evaluation

Initial assessment
- Vital signs, including orthostatics
- Check heart rate and rhythm
- Oxygen saturation
- Fingerstick blood glucose
- Assess level of consciousness

History
- Warning symptoms prior to fall
- Activity and location before fall
- Patient's perception of why he or she fell
- Details of fall from any witnesses
- History of previous falls
- History of hypoglycemia/diabetes
- Administration of any PRN medications, especially sedatives, low-potency neuroleptics, and tricyclic antidepressants
- Subjective experience of pain, including location and intensity
- Any perceived/witnessed loss of consciousness

(*Continued*)

	Examination
	Signs of volume depletion, including hydration status (skin turgor, oral moistness)
	Entire body for lacerations, bruises, and/or bleeds
	Mental status examination for signs of delirium and/or stupor
	Head for meningismus, cerebrospinal fluid (CSF) leak, raccoon eyes, Battles sign
	Fundi for papilledema or retinal hemorrhages
	Neurologic exam for sensory or motor deficits, gait and coordination
	Cardiologic examination for carotid bruits, irregular heartbeat, weak pulses
	Musculoskeletal examination to rule out fractures
Possible complications	Head injury
	Limb, hip, and wrist fractures
	Lacerations, bruises, and bleeds (especially in patients with chronic liver disease, history of alcoholism, antiplatelet/anticoagulant treatment)
Management	Studies
	Complete blood cell count (CBC) with differential, CHEM 7, Ca, Mg, PO4, hepatic function, urinalysis, toxicology screen, drug levels, cultures if indicated, stool guaiac, coagulation studies
	Other studies if indicated include EKG, x-rays of limb(s), brain imaging
	Treatment
	Manage contributory cause
	Address any sequelae of the fall, including lacerations (pressure, Derma bond, surgery consult as needed), fractures (immobilize limb or patient and page orthopedics)
	Rule out any covert coexisting etiologies, such as substance withdrawal/intoxication
	Prevention
	Safety precautions, such as call bell, 1:1 observation, call light
	Evaluate medication, particularly administration of sedating and hypotensive medications, timing, and dosing
	Identify patients in need of assistive devices and consider physical therapy referral
	For patients at repeated risk of harm due to volitional falls, consider safety devices such as padded helmets

References

Bernstein CA, Ladds BJ, Maloney AS, et al. *On Call Psychiatry*. Philadelphia: W.B. Saunders Company; 1997:154–157.

Green GB, Harris IS, Lin GA, et al., eds. *The Washington Manual of Medical Therapeutics*. 31st ed. Philadelphia: Lippincott Williams & Wilkins; 2004.

Chapter 13

FEVER

Differential Diagnosis of Fever

Infection	Bacterial
	  Meningitis, upper/lower respiratory infections (e.g., pneumonia, tuberculosis), endocarditis, cholecystitis, appendicitis, cellulitis, diverticulitis, upper and lower genitourinary infections
	Viral
	  Common cold, HIV, mononucleosis, hepatitis
	Fungal, rickettsial, parasitic

Collagen vascular disease	Rheumatoid arthritis, rheumatic fever, lupus, polyarteritis nodosa, sarcoidosis, temporal arteritis, vasculitis
Malignancy	Leukemia, lymphoma, renal cell carcinoma, hepatocellular carcinoma, lung cancer, pancreatic cancer
Medications	Anesthetics, antibiotics, anticholinergics, antipsychotics, lithium, steroids, tricyclic antidepressants, thyroid hormone, alcohol withdrawal
Central nervous system	Head trauma, mass lesions
Cardiovascular	Myocardial infarction, deep venous thrombosis, thrombophlebitis, pulmonary embolism
Gastrointestinal	Hepatitis, inflammatory bowel disease
Endocrine	Acute adrenal insufficiency, gout, thyroid storm, pheochromocytoma
Hyperthermia	Neuroleptic malignant syndrome, heat stroke, anesthetic hyperthermia
Psychiatric	Serotonin syndrome, factitious fever
Miscellaneous	Atelectasis, transfusion reaction, transplant rejection, tissue injury, hematoma, IV lines

Workup

- Complete history, including infectious contacts, travel, pets, occupation, medications, review of systems, past medical history, social history, tuberculosis history, intravenous (IV) drug use, immunosuppression or neutropenia, history of cancer.
- Elicit details such as timing and pattern of fever, as well as associated symptoms (e.g., localizing symptoms, cough, headache, shortness of breath, weight loss, joint pain, leg pain, urinary urgency).

- Assessment of vital signs, including rectal temperature, blood pressure, heart rate, respiratory rate, pulse oximetry, fingerstick blood glucose.
- Thorough physical exam with attention to skin findings, lymph node enlargement, murmurs, hepatosplenomegaly, presence of ascites, arthritis, inspection of all lines (e.g., IV lines, Foley catheter), wounds.
- Laboratory studies, including complete blood cell count (CBC) with differential, chemistry panel, hepatic function, erythrocyte sedimentation rate (ESR), antinuclear antibodies (ANA), rheumatoid factor (RF), blood cultures ×3 off antibiotics, urinalysis, urine culture, PPD skin test, HIV.
- Imaging studies as indicated based on workup and clinical findings, including chest x-ray, abdominal CT (oral and IV contrast), right upper quadrant (RUQ) ultrasound, lumbar puncture, brain imaging, temporal artery biopsy (if ESR elevated and age >60).

Management

- Consult medicine.
- Indications for hospitalization include temperature >104 degrees, hyperthermic syndrome, evidence of sepsis/bacteremia, patients who are elderly, immunocompromised and/or have comorbid medical illness, altered mental status, unstable vital signs.
- Discontinue unnecessary medications, infected lines.
- Consider antipyretics, such as aspirin/acetaminophen 325–650 mg p.o. q4–6h scheduled/prn fever.
- Empiric antibiotics typically not indicated unless patient neutropenic.
- Antibiotics administered when bacterial infection is identified and/or suspected in a high-risk patient.
- Refer to drug-induced neurologic syndromes in Psychiatry section for further guidance in workup and management of neuroleptic malignant syndrome and serotonin syndrome.

References

Green GB, Harris IS, Lin GA, et al., eds. *The Washington Manual of Medical Therapeutics*. 31st ed. Philadelphia: Lippincott Williams & Wilkins; 2004:293–294.

Manu P, Suarez RE, Barnett BJ, eds. *Handbook of Medicine in Psychiatry*. Arlington: American Psychiatric Publishing, Inc; 2006:21–31.

Sabatine MS, ed. *The Massachusetts General Hospital Handbook of Internal Medicine*. Philadelphia: Lippincott Williams & Wilkins; 2000:6–21.

Tierney LM, McPhee SJ, Papadakis MA. *2006 Current Medical Diagnosis and Treatment*. 45th ed. New York: McGraw-Hill Companies, Inc; 2006:26–27.

Chapter 14

VIRAL HEPATITIS

Type	Transmission	Risk Factors	Serologies
Hepatitis A	Fecal–oral	Contaminated food and water Children and caregivers in daycare centers	**Acute** IgM anti-HAV+ **Chronic** N/A **Recovered/latent** IgG anti-HAV+ **Vaccinated** IgG anti-HAV+
Hepatitis B	Blood Percutaneous Sexual Perinatal	Intravenous drug users Unsafe sexual practices Infants born to infected mothers Health care workers Transfusion recipients	**Acute** HBsAg+ IgM anti-HBc+ HBeAg+ HBV DNA+ **Chronic** IgG anti-HBc+ HBeAg+/− (present during periods of high replication) Anti-HBe+/− (present during periods of low replication) HBsAg+ HBV DNA +/− (present during periods of high replication) **Recovered/latent** IgG anti-HBc+ HBV DNA− HBeAg− Anti-HBe+/− HBsAg− Anti-HBs+ **Vaccinated** Anti-HBs+ only
Hepatitis C	Blood Percutaneous Sexual (rare) Perinatal (rare)	Intravenous drug users Transfusion recipients	**Acute** All tests possibly negative HCV RNA+ Anti-HCV Ab+ in 8–10 weeks

(*Continued*)

Type	Transmission	Risk Factors	Serologies
			Chronic Anti-HCV Ab+ HCV RNA+ **Recovered/latent** Anti-HCV Ab+ HCV RNA− **Vaccinated** N/A
Hepatitis D	Blood Sexual (rare)	Any person with hepatitis B Intravenous drug users	Positive hepatitis B serologies plus the following: **Acute** IgM anti-HDV+ HDV Ag+ **Chronic** IgG anti-HDV+ **Recovered/latent** IgG anti-HDV+ **Vaccinated** N/A
Hepatitis E	Fecal–oral	Contaminated food and water Travel to endemic regions	IgM anti-HEV through Centers for Disease Control (CDC)

Adapted from Green GB, Harris IS, Lin GA, et al., eds. *The Washington Manual of Medical Therapeutics*. 31st ed. Philadelphia: Lippincott Williams & Wilkins; 2004:382, with permission.

Psychiatric Implications of Comorbid Hepatitis C

- Interferon—insidious onset of cognitive impairment, depression (~20% to 40%), irritability (20% to 30%), anxiety disorders (~10% to 20%), insomnia (40%), fatigue (70%), psychosis (<5%) that typically are unpredictable and potentially lethal (e.g., suicidality).
- Interferon-induced impulsivity and hostility may increase the risk of dangerous behavior and suicide attempts.
- Psychiatric effects of interferon may be reversible with significant dose reduction.
- Comorbid substance abuse is prevalent and requires intervention to avoid exacerbation of hepatitis and psychiatric illness.
- Chronic viral hepatitis does not preclude the use of hepatotoxic medications but close monitoring is required and the medication must be stopped if the patient has rising liver function test values.

Management Considerations for Comorbid Hepatitis C

- Close coordination with primary care provider and gastroenterologist/hepatologist.

- Prior to initiating therapy with interferon/ribavirin, assess the following:
  - Presence of neuropsychiatric symptoms, including severity.
  - Suicidality.
  - If the patient has weapons, arrange for removal prior to initiating therapy.
  - Presence of comorbid substance use and past psychiatric history.
  - Baseline thyroid stimulating hormone (TSH).
  - Educate significant others about the risks and warning signs of worsening psychiatric symptoms.
- During therapy with interferon/ribavirin:
  - Close and careful monitoring of neuropsychiatric symptoms, including detailed documentation to enable serial assessment of severity and progression of symptoms.
  - Continuous monitoring of suicide risk, including access to weapons.
  - When indicated, consider treatment of depression with selective serotonin reuptake inhibitors (SSRIs) with fewer cytochrome P450 drug interactions (e.g., citalopram, escitalopram). Ensure bipolar disorder is ruled out prior to antidepressant treatment.

References

Bourgeois JA. Depression as co-pilot: clinical implications of hepatitis C and interferon/ribavirin treatment. *Psychiatr Times.* 12(5):18–19.

Goff DC, Medical morbidity and mortality in schizophrenia: guidelines for psychiatrists. *J Clin Psychiatr.* 66(2):183–192.

Green GB, Harris IS, Lin GA, et al., eds. *The Washington Manual of Medical Therapeutics.* 31st ed. Philadelphia: Lippincott Williams & Wilkins; 2004:380–386.

Henry C, Castera L, Demotes-Mainard J. Hepatitis C and interferon: watch for hostility, impulsivity. *Curr Psychiatr.* 5(8):71–77.

Sabatine MS, ed. *The Massachusetts General Hospital Handbook of Internal Medicine.* Philadelphia: Lippincott Williams & Wilkins; 2000:3-16–3-17.

Chapter 15

HUMAN BITE

Pathogens	Streptococci
	Staphylococci
	Fusobacterium spp.
	Eikenella corrodens
Evaluation	Record mechanism of injury (such as closed fist)
	Assess location, depth, size, and type of wound
	Evidence of infection, including redness, lymph node involvement, discharge
	Factors indicating a high-risk bite wound include location (on hands, genitalia, or near joints), puncture or crush wounds vs lacerations, and compromised immune status
Management	Moderate to severe wounds, presence of infection, and/or other high-risk factors warrant medicine consultation
	Management includes copious irrigation, topical antimicrobial, dressing as indicated, wound elevation, tetanus booster (if not administered in the last 5 years), pain management, and suturing for facial wounds
	Studies may include cultures from visibly infected wounds and x-rays to rule out fracture, foreign body, and/or joint space involvement.
	Antimicrobial treatment is indicated for evidence of infection and prophylaxis of high-risk bite wounds and may include amoxicillin/clavulanate 875 mg/125 mg p.o. BID for 3–5 d for uninfected wounds
	Infected wounds/bone and/or joint involvement require intravenous therapy and medicine consultation

References

Green GB, Harris IS, Lin GA, et al., eds. *The Washington Manual of Medical Therapeutics*. 31st ed. Philadelphia: Lippincott Williams & Wilkins; 2004:320.

Chapter 16

HYPERTENSION

General Considerations

- Primary/essential hypertension—95% of all hypertension with no primary etiology identified.
- Secondary hypertension—5% secondary to causes including renal disease and endocrine disorders, among others.
- Elevated blood pressures should be based on two readings separated by 2 min, with verification of measurement in the contralateral arm.
- Close coordination with primary care provider for appropriate evaluation and management of elevated blood pressures. Evaluation may entail obtaining the following information:
  - Personal and family history of cardiovascular, cerebrovascular, or renal disease, and/or diabetes mellitus.
  - Diet, sodium intake, drug use (e.g., smoking, alcohol), nutrition, medications (e.g., oral contraceptives).
  - Comprehensive physical examination, including fundoscopic and neurologic.
  - Studies including chemistry panel, Ca, Mg, PO_4, complete blood cell count (CBC), urinalysis, lipid profile, EKG, chest x-ray.

Classification and Initial Management of Blood Pressure in Adults

Hypertension	Systolic Blood Pressure (mm Hg)	Diastolic Blood Pressure (mm Hg)	Lifestyle Modification	Pharmacotherapy Considerations
Normal	<120	And <80	Encourage	N/A
Prehypertension	120–139	Or 80–89	Yes	No antihypertensive drug indicated.
Stage 1 hypertension	140–159	Or 90–99	Yes	Thiazide-like diuretics and beta-blockers for most. May consider angiotensin-converting enzyme inhibitor, angiotensin receptor blocker, calcium channel blocker, or combination.
Stage II hypertension	≥160	Or ≥100	Yes	2-drug therapy for most.
Hypertensive urgency	≥210	Or ≥120 and asymptomatic with minimal or no end organ damage	N/A	Reduce blood pressure over 24–48 h using oral agents.
Hypertensive emergency	≥180	Or ≥110 and symptomatic/presence of end organ damage	N/A	Reduce blood pressure with IV antihypertensives and transfer immediately to emergency room.

Adapted from Chobanian AV, et al. The Seventh Report of the Joint National Committee on Prevention, Detection, Evaluation, and Treatment of High Blood Pressure: the JNC 7 report. *JAMA*. 2003;289:25–60.

Lifestyle Modifications

- Reduce weight to maintain body mass index between 18.5 and 25.
- Stop alcohol and cigarette smoking.
- Dietary restrictions, including decreasing saturated fat, low cholesterol diet, reducing sodium intake to 2.4 g per day (6 g of sodium).
- Increase aerobic physical activity (30–45 min most days of the week).
- Strict glucose control in diabetes mellitus.
- Regular follow-up with primary care provider.

Pharmacotherapy Considerations for Hypertension

Drugs by Class	Example Antihypertensive[a]	Initial Dosage	Adverse Effects	Special Considerations for Class
Diuretics	Hydrochlorthiazide	12.5–25 mg p.o. qd	Electrolyte disturbances, increased glucose, LDL and triglycerides, rash, erectile dysfunction, muscle weakness.	Indicated first-line agents for uncomplicated hypertension. Beneficial in patients with comorbid heart failure.
Beta-blockers	Atenolol Metoprolol	25–50 mg p.o. qd 50 mg in 1 or 2 divided doses	Bronchospasm, sinus node dysfunction, atrioventricular defect, worsening of left ventricular failure, depression, fatigue, lethargy, impotence.	Drugs of choice for preexisting coronary artery disease. Contraindicated in stimulant use.
Calcium-channel blockers	Amlodipine Nifedipine	5 mg p.o. qd 30 mg p.o. qd	Edema, dizziness, palpitations, headache, hypotension, worsening of heart failure.	May exacerbate and/or cause heart failure in patients with preexisting cardiac dysfunction.
Angiotensin-converting enzyme inhibitors	Benazepril Lisinopril	10 mg p.o. qd 5–10 mg p.o. qd	Cough, hypotension, dizziness, renal dysfunction, hyperkalemia, angioedema, altered taste, rash.	Requires monitoring of K and Cr. Contraindicated in pregnancy. May be drug of choice for diabetes mellitus and heart failure.
Angiotensin-II receptor blockers	Valsartan	80 mg p.o. qd	Hyperkalemia, renal dysfunction. Rarely, angioedema.	Requires monitoring of K and Cr. Contraindicated in pregnancy.
Alpha-adrenergic blockers	Prazosin	1 mg p.o. qd	Syncope, postural hypotension, dizziness, palpitations, headache, weakness, sexual dysfunction, anticholinergic effects, urinary incontinence.	Decreased risk of syncope/presyncope with bedtime dosing, gradual titration, and repeated use.
Centrally acting adrenergic agents	Clonidine	0.1 mg p.o. twice daily	Sedation, dry mouth, sexual dysfunction, headache, constipation.	Rebound hypertension with sudden discontinuation. Risk of heart failure in patients with decreased left ventricular function.
Vasodilators	Hydralazine	25 mg p.o. twice daily	Gastrointestinal disturbances, tachycardia, postural hypotension, headache, rash, lupus-like syndrome.	May worsen and/or precipitate angina/ischemic heart disease.

[a] Example antihypertensives provided are not all-inclusive. Choice of antihypertensive varies from patient to patient.

Hypertensive Emergency
Definition
- Systolic blood pressure (BP) ≥180 or diastolic ≥110 plus end organ damage associated with any *one* of the following:
  - Neurological damage—encephalopathy, papilledema, stroke.
  - Cardiac damage—unstable angina or acute myocardial infarct (MI), heart failure with pulmonary edema, aortic dissection.
  - Renal damage—acute renal failure, proteinurea, hematuria.
  - Microangiopathic hemolytic anemia.
  - Preeclampsia-eclampsia.

Warning Signs
- Headache
- Visual changes
- Change in mental status/encephalopathy
- Chest pain
- Shortness of breath

Conditions to Consider When Presenting in the Psychiatric Unit
- Cocaine, methamphetamine, LSD, PCP intoxication.
- Drug overdose, including anticholinergic intoxication.
- Drug withdrawal, including alcohol and sedative-hypnotic withdrawal.
- Drug interactions, such as monamine oxidase inhibitors with tyramine-containing foods, rebound hypertension from discontinuation of antihypertensives (e.g., clonidine, angiotensin-converting enzyme inhibitor).
- Psychotropic-induced syndromes, including neuroleptic, malignant, and serotonin syndromes.

Management
- Requires control of blood pressure with IV antihypertensives and immediate transfer to the emergency unit/intensive care unit.
- Check blood pressure every 15–30 min, monitor closely until patient is transferred.
- Initial management may involve a focused history and physical examination.
- Initial studies may include chemistry panel, Ca, Mg, PO4, CBC with differential, urinalysis, toxicology screen, arterial blood gases, EKG, chest x-ray.
- Excessive or rapid decreases in blood pressure should be avoided to minimize the risk of cerebral hypoperfusion or coronary insufficiency.

Management of Hypertensive Urgency
Definition
- Systolic BP ≥210 or diastolic ≥120 with minimal or no end organ damage in an asymptomatic patient.

Management

- Coordinate care with primary care provider/inpatient medicine team.
- May be controlled with increased doses of oral antihypertensives and close monitoring.
- Recheck blood pressure in 1 h and evaluate closely for presence of signs and symptoms of end organ damage.

References

Chobanian AV, The Seventh Report of the Joint National Committee on Prevention, Detection, Evaluation, and Treatment of High Blood Pressure: the JNC 7 report. *JAMA.* 2003;289:25–60.

Green GB, Harris IS, Lin GA, et al., eds. *The Washington Manual of Medical Therapeutics.* 31st ed. Philadelphia: Lippincott Williams & Wilkins; 2004:76–89.

Manu P, Suarez RE, Barnett BJ, eds. *Handbook of Medicine in Psychiatry.* Arlington: American Psychiatric Publishing, Inc; 2006:33–39.

Rosen H. *The Consult Manual of Internal Medicine.* Med Consult Publishing, Inc; 2006:60–75.

Sabatine MS, ed. *The Massachusetts General Hospital Handbook of Internal Medicine.* Philadelphia: Lippincott Williams & Wilkins; 2000:1-29–1-30.

Tierney LM, McPhee SJ, Papadakis MA. *2006 Current Medical Diagnosis and Treatment.* 45th ed. New York: McGraw-Hill Companies, Inc; 2006:420–438.

Chapter 17

THYROID DISORDERS

	Hypothyroidism	Hyperthyroidism

Common causes	Primary (e.g, Hashimoto disease)
	Secondary (e.g., disorders of pituitary or hypothalamus)
	Iatrogenic (e.g., thyroidectomy, radioactive iodine therapy)
	Inflammation—thyroiditis (e.g., postpartum)
	Drug-induced
	  Lithium
	  Glucocorticoids
		Graves disease
		Inflammation—thyroiditis
		Toxic multinodular goiter
		Neoplastic—adenomas
		Factitious hyperthyroidism

Clinical features	Depression Weakness Fatigue Cold intolerance Somnolence Impaired memory Headache Constipation Menorrhagia Myalgia Hoarseness Paresthesias	Anxiety Heat intolerance Weight loss Weakness Palpitations Oligomenorrhea Diarrhea
Exam findings	Hair thinning Facial and periorbital edema Presence or absence of goiter Dry skin Thin, brittle nails Delayed deep tendon reflexes Bradycardia Non-pitting edema (myxedema) Mild weight gain Rare hypoventilation, pericardial or pleural effusions, deafness, carpal tunnel syndrome	Eyelid lag Stare Goiter/nodules Proximal weakness Brisk deep tendon reflexes Fine tremor Tachycardia/atrial fibrillation Exacerbation of coronary artery disease Warm, moist skin

Diagnostic findings	Primary hypothyroidism
	  Elevated TSH
	  Decreased free T4
	Secondary hypothyroidism
	  Plasma TSH may be within reference levels
	Other potential findings may include hyponatremia, anemia, elevated lipids, elevated liver
		Decreased TSH
		Elevated free T4 and/or T3

(*Continued*)

	Hypothyroidism	Hyperthyroidism
	enzymes, elevated creatine kinase Of note, many illnesses (e.g., acute psychiatric illness, starvation, autoimmune disease, trauma, surgery, severe illness) can alter thyroid tests without causing thyroid dysfunction	
Management	Consult and coordinate care with endocrinology. Treatment may entail the following: T4 (levothyroxine) replacement at doses 50–150 mcg daily taken before a meal (lower in elderly and in patients with cardiac disease). Rule out adrenal insufficiency before starting thyroid hormone replacement therapy.	Consult and coordinate care with endocrinology. Treatment may entail symptomatic therapy (e.g., beta-adrenergic antagonist), propylthiouracil/methimazole, radioactive iodine, subtotal thyroidectomy. Urgent intervention is especially required in the setting of exacerbation of heart disease, associated fever, delirium, comorbid medical illness, pregnancy.

References

Green GB, Harris IS, Lin GA, et al., eds. *The Washington Manual of Medical Therapeutics*. 31st ed. Philadelphia: Lippincott Williams & Wilkins; 2004:488–496.

Manu P, Suarez RE, Barnett BJ, eds. *Handbook of Medicine in Psychiatry*. Arlington: American Psychiatric Publishing, Inc; 2006:435–443.

Rosen H. *The Consult Manual of Internal Medicine*. Med Consult Publishing; 2006:386–398.

Sabatine MS, ed. *The Massachusetts General Hospital Handbook of Internal Medicine*. Philadelphia: Lippincott Williams & Wilkins; 2000. 7–3 to 7–5.

Tierney LM, McPhee SJ, Papadakis MA. *2006 Current Medical Diagnosis and Treatment*. 45th ed. New York: McGraw-Hill Companies, Inc; 2006:1131–1133, 1135–1143.

Chapter 18

METABOLIC SYNDROME

Three or more of the following risk factors are required for the National Cholesterol Education Program (NCEP) Adult Treatment Panel (ATP) III criteria.

Risk Factor	Defining Level
Abdominal obesity	Waist circumference (at umbilicus)
Men	>102 cm (>40 in.)
Women	>88 cm (>35 in.)
Triglycerides	≥150 mg/dL
HDL cholesterol	
Men	<40 mg/dL
Women	<50 mg/dL
Blood pressure	≥130/≥85 mm Hg
Fasting glucose	≥110 mg/dL

Reprinted from Janicak PG. Major mental disorders and the metabolic syndrome. A *Supplement to Current Psychiatry*. December 2004:4, with permission.

Mental Illness and the Metabolic Syndrome

- Risk factors contributing to the development of metabolic syndrome include poor nutrition, sedentary lifestyle, comorbid substance use, social isolation, financial hardship, noncompliance, limited access to medical care, decreased ability to care for self.
- Treatment with psychiatric medications can cause and/or worsen these risk factors for metabolic syndrome.
  - Weight gain—clozapine, olanzapine > risperidone, quetiapine > aripiprazole, ziprasidone.
  - Risk for diabetes mellitus and lipid abnormalities—clozapine and olanzapine increased risk, aripiprazole and ziprasidone no known risk, olanzapine and risperidone unclear risk.

Psychotropic-Medication Induced Weight Gain

May Cause Significant Weight Gain	May Cause Little or No Weight Gain (or Weight Loss)
Antidepressants	Antidepressants
Paroxetine, other SSRIs	Bupropion
Mirtazapine	
MAOIs, TCAs	
Anticonvulsants	Anticonvulsants
Valproate	Topiramate

(*Continued*)

May Cause Significant Weight Gain	May Cause Little or No Weight Gain (or Weight Loss)
Carbamazepine	Lamotrigine
Gabapentin	Zonisamide
Antipsychotics	Antipsychotics
Most	Ziprasidone
Clozapine	Aripiprazole
Olanzapine	
Moderate	
Risperidone	
Quetiapine	
Lithium	

SSRIs, selective serotonin reuptake inhibitors; MAOIs, monoamine oxidase inhibitors; TCAs, tricyclic antidepressants.
Modified from Janicak PG. Major mental disorders and the metabolic syndrome. *A Supplement to Current Psychiatry.* December 2004:10.

Management Principles

- Counsel patient on the risks/benefits of introducing psychiatric medications that can worsen and/or exacerbate risk factors for metabolic syndrome.
- Document baseline assessment of and continue to monitor values for body mass index, waist circumference, blood pressure, fasting plasma glucose, fasting lipids. See Section IV, Chapter 50 on physical health monitoring.
- Identify patients at increased risk for metabolic syndrome.
- Continue to reevaluate psychotropic regimen ensuring stability of the patient's mental illness while minimizing adverse effects, risk factors for metabolic syndrome, and polypharmacy.
- Encourage lifestyle modifications, such as increased physical activity, improved nutrition, and decreasing comorbid substance use.
- Close coordination with primary care provider, including referral for further evaluation and management when metabolic syndrome is suspected. Ensure thorough assessment is performed to rule out medical etiologies for dyslipidemia, obesity (e.g., hypothyroidism), and hypertension.
- Consider referrals when indicated to chemical dependency programs and nutrition counseling.

References

Janicak PG. Major mental disorders and the metabolic syndrome. *A Supplement to Current Psychiatry.* December 2004:3–11.
Nasrallah HA. Metabolic findings from the CATIE Trial and their relation to tolerability. *CNS Spectrums: Int J Neuropsychiatr Med.* 2006;11(7) (suppl 7):32–39.

Chapter 19

NAUSEA AND VOMITING

Differential Diagnosis of Nausea and Vomiting

Gastrointestinal	Obstruction/pseudo-obstruction
	Inflammation/infection—appendicitis, peritonitis, pancreatitis, acute cholecystitis, viral and bacterial gastroenteritis (*Staphylococcus aureas, Bacillus cereus, Clostridium perfingens*), ingested poisons or toxins
	Gastroparesis (functional gastric outlet obstruction)
	Small intestinal dysmotility
Cardiovascular	Congestive heart failure
	Acute myocardial infarction
Metabolic/endocrine	Diabetic ketoacidosis
	Addison disease
	Hypo/hyperthyroidism
	Pregnancy
	Hepatic disease
	Hypercalcemia
Central nervous system	Head injury
	Meningitis
	Headache
	Vestibular disorder (e.g., Ménière disease, tumor)
Renal	Nephrolithiasis
	End stage renal disease
Medications	Lithium
	Selective serotonin reuptake inhibitors
	Valproic acid
	Venlafaxine
	Anticholinergic agents
	Nefazodone
	Narcotics
	Digitalis
	Digoxin
	Oral contraceptive agents
Psychiatric	Anorexia
	Bulimia nervosa
	Depressive disorders
	Anxiety disorders
	Irritable bowel syndrome
	Somatoform disorders (e.g., somatization, factitious disorders, malingering)

Workup Considerations
- Acute
  - Gastrointestinal infections
  - Food poisoning
  - Drug ingestion
  - Obstruction
  - Perforation
- Chronic
  - Drug ingestion
  - Metabolic disorders
  - Progressive, partial obstruction
  - Motility disorders
- Early morning vomiting
  - Increased intracranial pressure
  - Anxiety
  - Pregnancy
  - Alcoholism
  - Uremia
- Vomiting of psychogenic origin (e.g., anorexia, bulimia, psychotic and delusional states)
  - Occurs during or immediately after a meal
  - Is generally never public
- Intestinal obstruction
  - Copious
  - Bilious (if bilious, obstruction is distal to the pylorus), fecal odor
  - No passage of flatus in incomplete obstruction
- Bloody emesis
  - Esophageal, gastric, or intestinal inflammation
  - Esophageal, gastric, or intestinal malignancy
  - Alcoholism (e.g., esophageal varices)
  - Mallory–Weiss syndrome

Assessment
- History, including patient's psychiatric diagnosis, comorbid medical conditions, current medications, recent substance use
- Associated signs and symptoms, such as
  - Abdominal, chest, back, rectal pain
  - Obstipation
  - Diarrhea
  - Nature of the emesis (bright red blood, dark blood with clots, coffee grounds, bilious, fecal odor, undigested food)
  - Rough estimate of the volume of the emesis and the frequency
  - Passage of flatus
- Vital signs
- General evaluation, including anemia, jaundice, mucosal pigmentation, lymphadenopathy, hernia, hand examination (e.g., ulceration indicative of self-induced vomiting), loss of dental enamel
- Cardiovascular—signs of congestive heart failure

- Abdominal examination
  - Peritoneal signs (abdominal distension, involuntary guarding, tenderness, lack of bowel sounds), palpable masses require an urgent surgical consult
- Neurologic exam
  - Presence of focal deficits, papilledema, neck stiffness require neurologic consult

Management

- Studies may entail complete blood cell count (CBC) with differential, chemistry panel, serum blood levels, including lithium, depakote, toxicology screen, urine pregnancy test, hepatic function, amylase, lipase, EKG, brain imaging as indicated
- If unable to determine etiology, transfer to surgery/medicine
- May be necessary to withhold oral intake or limit to clear liquids
- Do not prescribe antiemetics until the etiology of the vomiting is certain.
- Be sure that you have ruled out etiologies that pose a major threat to the patient's life as patients may have stable vital signs in some cases and etiologies
- Correct any significant electrolyte disturbances promptly
- In the case of psychiatric drug-induced vomiting decrease the dose or taper off
- If an eating disorder is suspected, consider meal watches (extending one hour after completing meals), supervised visits to bathroom, weighing each morning
- Antiemetics may be indicated (metoclopramide, promethazine, prochlorperazine) but only after etiology of nausea and vomiting is known. Consider the interactions of these medications on the patient's drug regimen before prescribing them

References

Manu P, Suarez RE, Barnett BJ, eds. *Handbook of Medicine in Psychiatry.* Arlington: American Psychiatric Publishing, Inc; 2006:223–230.

Tierney LM, McPhee SJ, Papadakis MA. *2006 Current Medical Diagnosis and Treatment.* 45th ed. New York: McGraw-Hill Companies, Inc; 2006:538–540.

Chapter 20

TUBERCULOSIS SCREENING

Screening	High-risk individuals
	Immunocompromised individuals (particularly HIV positive)
	Immigrants from high prevalence countries
	Malnourished, homeless, and those living in overcrowded and substandard housing
	Alcoholics
	IV drug users
	Chronic systemic illness, such as diabetes
	Residents of long-term care facilities, including nursing homes and prisons
	Ongoing potential contact with cases of active TB, such as health care providers and prison guards
	Exceptions to annual screening
	Documented positive TB skin test in the past
	Prior treatment of a positive TB skin test
Skin testing	Administer Mantoux test (0.1 ml of purified protein derivative [PPD] containing 5 tuberculin units)
	Read 48–72 h later
	Measure induration, not erythema
	Measurement should be one number that is measured in the greatest transverse plane

Classification of positive PPD	PPD induration	Group
	≥5mm	HIV-positive persons
		Recent contact with individuals with active TB
		Chest x-ray changes consistent with old, healed TB
		Patients with suppressed immune systems
	≥10 mm	Patients who are non-immunosuppressed, with the risk factors above
		Children and adolescents exposed to adults at high risk
		TB skin test converters (increase of) >10 mm induration within a 2-year period
	≥15 mm	All other persons

Limitations	False positive
	Previous BCG vaccination
	Infection with nontuberculous mycobacteria
	False negative
	Patients who are immunocompromised
	Recent infection (1.5–3 months required to develop adequate cellular immunity)
Treatment considerations	Rule out active TB using chest x-ray, symptom review, and/or sputum collection

(Continued)

- Once active TB is ruled out, administer INH 300 mg p.o. qd ×9 months for chemoprophylaxis. Perform baseline hepatic function testing and neurologic examination prior to initiating INH treatment and monthly thereafter. Pyridoxine 10 mg p.o. qd may be given concurrently as prophylaxis for neuritis
- INH is contraindicated in active liver disease and pregnancy
- Referral to the health department for chemoprophylaxis is recommended to ensure adherence and to monitor for medication-related side effects
- All suspected and confirmed cases of tuberculosis should be reported promptly to local and state public health authorities
- Referral to appropriate agencies and specialists for further management should be made when active disease is detected/suspected

References

Green GB, Harris IS, Lin GA, et al., eds. *The Washington Manual of Medical Therapeutics*. 31st ed. Philadelphia: Lippincott Williams & Wilkins; 2004:307–309.

Okoye O, Ravakhah. Tuberculin skin testing: methods and indications. *Resident Staff Physician*. 2005;51(10):40–43.

Rosen H. *The Consult Manual of Internal Medicine*. Med Consult Publishing Inc; 2006:603–610.

Tierney LM, McPhee SJ, Papadakis MA. *2006 Current Medical Diagnosis and Treatment*. 45th ed. New York: McGraw-Hill Companies, Inc; 2006:256–263.

Chapter 21

SMOKING CESSATION PHARMACOTHERAPY

General Considerations

- Common side effects for nicotine therapy may include headache, insomnia, nightmares, nausea, dizziness, and blurred vision.
- Nicotine use may be contraindicated during pregnancy and lactation, in patients with coronary artery disease (particularly 2 weeks post myocardial infarction, worsening angina), peripheral vascular disease, serious arrhythmias, allergy to nicotine. Weigh risks and benefits prior to administration.
- Refer to package insert for further treatment recommendations depending on formulation available, as well as other potential precautions and adverse effects.

Pharmacotherapy

1. Bupropion SR (Zyban): Antidepressant with dopaminergic and adrenergic properties.
   - Dose 150 mg p.o. qd for 3 d and then increase to 150 mg p.o. BID for 7–12 weeks.
   - Set quit date for 1–2 weeks after beginning treatment.
   - Side effects may include dry mouth, insomnia, agitation, and seizures, in approximately 0.1% to 0.4% of patients.
   - Contraindicated in eating disorders, history of seizures.
   - Longer duration recommended to improve long-term cessation rates.
2. Transdermal nicotine patches.
   - Nicotine transdermal patch (>10 cigarettes per day): 21-mg patch qd ×4–8 weeks, 14-mg patch qd ×2–4 weeks, 7-mg patch qd ×2–4 weeks.
   - Nicotrol (>10 cigarettes per day): 15-mg patch every 16 h ×4 weeks, 10-mg patch every 16 h ×2 weeks, 5-mg patch every 16 h ×2 weeks.
   - Side effects may include redness and pruritus at the patch site, which may respond to topical steroid cream.
3. Nicotine nasal spray (Nicotrol NS).
   - One (0.5 mg) spray to each nostril q1–2 h. Maximum 5 sprays per hour or 40 doses per day (for heavier smokers).
   - Delivers nicotine more rapidly than a gum, patch, or inhaler but less rapidly than a cigarette.
   - Side effects may include sneezing, excess lacrimation, and cough.
   - Nasal irritation occurs in majority of users and typically does not improve.
4. Nicotine inhaler (Nicotrol inhaler).
   - One (10 mg per cartridge) is used over 20 min.

- Six to sixteen cartridges per day for 12 weeks, followed by tapering over 6 to 12 weeks.
- Side effects may also include cough and irritation of the mouth.
5. Nicotine gum (Nicorette).
    - 2-mg or 4-mg pieces (up to 60 mg per day).
    - Start with one piece every 1 to 2 h then gradually taper.
    - Avoid food and drink 15 min prior to and during use.
6. Nicotine lozenges.
    - 2-mg lozenge used q1–2 h prn, not to exceed 20 lozenges over 24 h.
7. Combination therapy.
    - Several studies indicate improved efficacy and decreased cravings in heavy smokers when bupropion is administered concurrently with a nicotine patch compared to a nicotine patch alone.
    - Additionally, heavy smokers may require concurrent treatment with long- and short-acting nicotine replacement agents.

References

Green GB, Harris IS, Lin GA, et al., eds. *The Washington Manual of Medical Therapeutics*. 31st ed. Philadelphia: Lippincott Williams & Wilkins; 2004:222–223.

Tierney LM, McPhee SJ, Papadakis MA. *2006 Current Medical Diagnosis and Treatment*. 45th ed. New York: McGraw-Hill Companies, Inc; 2006:9.

Chapter 22

URINALYSIS

Urine Finding	Interpretation
Specific gravity	Workup of polyuria, acute renal failure, and rapid estimate of urine osmolarity.
pH	Normal 4.5–8.5 Workup of renal tubular acidosis, etiologic organisms for urinary tract infection (if >7 consider urea splitters, proteus, pseudomonas, klebsiella), stone disease and management of conditions where urinary alkalinization is required (rhabdomyolysis, salicylate, NSAID overdose).
Protein	Causes for proteinuria (low grade: 1–2 g/day; nephrotic range: 3.5 g/day) Glomerular (disruption of barrier): glomerulonephritis, nephritic syndrome. Tubulointerstitial (reduced resorption of freely filtered protein): acute tubular necrosis, acute interstitial nephritis, Fanconi syndrome. Overflow (Increased production of freely filtered protein): multiple myeloma, acute myeloid leukemia. Functional: fever, stress, exercise, orthostatic (only when upright), congestive heart failure.
Leukocyte esterase/nitrites	Suggestive but not diagnostic for bacteriuria.
Glucose	If positive, assess for diabetes mellitus.
Ketones	Potential etiologies include fasting, post exercise states, pregnancy, diabetes mellitus.
Bilirubin	Increased in hemolytic processes and hepatocellular disease. Decreased with biliary obstruction and broad spectrum antibiotic use.
White blood cell count (WBC)	5 leukocytes per high-power field = significant pyuria. May indicate infection but other causes include calculous disease, strictures, neoplasm, and glomerulonephropathy.
Red blood cell count (RBC)	5 erythrocytes per high-power field = significant hematuria. Presence of hematuria on dipstick and microscopic urinalysis requires workup.
Epithelial cells	Presence of squamous epithelial cells in the urinary sediment indicates contamination and warrants a repeat urine collection.

(*Continued*)

Urine Finding	Interpretation
	Large numbers of transitional epithelial cells may indicate possible neoplasm.
Casts	RBC casts: glomerular disease or vasculitis.
	WBC casts: pyelonephritis.
	Tubular casts: acute tubular nephritis.
	Hyaline casts: concentrated urine devoid of cells.
	Waxy casts: advanced renal failure, indicates stasis.
	Granular casts: any tubular injury.
	Pigmented casts: hemoglobin, myoglobin, bilirubin.
Crystals	Low pH: calcium oxalate, uric acid, cysteine.
	High pH: phosphate, struvite.
Bacteria and yeasts	Presence of organisms likely implies infection and must be confirmed by culture.

References

Sabatine MS, ed. *The Massachusetts General Hospital Handbook of Internal Medicine.* Philadelphia: Lippincott Williams & Wilkins; 2000:4–13.

Tierney LM, McPhee SJ, Papadakis MA. *2006 Current Medical Diagnosis and Treatment.* 45th ed. New York: McGraw-Hill Companies, Inc; 2006:934–935.

Chapter 23

URINARY TRACT INFECTIONS

Infection	Clinical Features	Treatment
Cystitis		
Uncomplicated cystitis: women who are not pregnant, without underlying structural or neurologic disease. Complicated cystitis: upper tract infection or any urinary tract infection in men or pregnant women or urinary tract infection with underlying structural or neurologic disease.	Pain on urination Urgency Increased frequency Change in urine color or odor Suprapubic pain	Uncomplicated: Trimethoprim/ sulfamethoxazole 160/800 mg 2 p.o. ×1 Ciprofloxacin 250 mg to 500 mg p.o. every 12 h ×3 d Ofloxacin 200 mg p.o. every 12 h ×3 d Complicated: Administer antibiotic regimens above ×10–14 d
Urethritis	Pain on urination Urgency Increased frequency Change in urine color or odor Suprapubic pain Urethral discharge	Treat for both *Neisseria* and *Chlamydia* *Neisseria:* ceftriaxone 125 mg IM ×1 Cefixime 400 mg p.o. ×1 *Chlamydia:* doxycycline 100 mg p.o. every 12 h ×7 d Azithromycin 1 g p.o. ×1
Prostatitis	Pain on urination Urgency Increased frequency Change in urine color or odor Suprapubic pain Sensation of incomplete emptying Weak stream	Acute Trimethoprim/ sulfamethoxazole 160/800 mg p.o. every 12 h ×21 d Ciprofloxacin 750 mg p.o. every 12 h ×21 d Ofloxacin 200–300 mg p.o. every 12 h ×21 d Chronic Trimethoprim/ sulfamethoxazole 160/ 800 mg p.o. every 12 h ×1–3 months Ciprofloxacin 250–500 mg p.o. every 12 h ×1–3 months Ofloxacin 200–400 mg p.o. every 12 h ×1–3 months

(*Continued*)

Infection	Clinical Features	Treatment

Pyelonephritis	Fever
	Shaking chills
	Flank or back pain
	Nausea
	Vomiting
	Diarrhea
		Acute
		Trimethoprim/
		  sulfamethoxazole
		  160/800 mg p.o.
		  every 12 h ×21 d
		Ciprofloxacin 750 mg
		  p.o. every 12 h ×21 d
		Ofloxacin 200–300 mg
		  every 12 h ×21 d
		Complicated cases may
		  require IV antibiotics

Diagnostic Considerations

- Urinalysis, both dipstick and microscopic.
  - Presence of pyuria (>8 leukocytes per high-power field) + bacteriuria (>1 organism per oil immersion field) +/− hematuria.
- Urine Gram stain and culture from clean catch midstream or straight catheterized specimen.
- Significant bacterial counts on culture.
  - $>10^5$ CFU/ml in asymptomatic women.
  - $>10^3$ CFU/ml in men.
  - $>10^2$ CFU/ml in symptomatic or catheterized patients.
- Refer to Chapter 22 on urinalysis.
- Further evaluation may entail blood cultures, screening for asymptomatic bacteriuria (e.g., pregnant women), cultures for *Chlamydia trachomatis* and *Neisseria gonorrhoeae*.

General Management Considerations

- For complicated infections, severe cases of urinary tract infections, pregnancy (e.g., avoid fluoroquinolones and tetracycline), and comorbid illnesses (e.g., diabetes mellitus), consult medicine.
- For pregnant women, explore teratogenic potential of antibiotics before administration.

References

Sabatine MS, ed. *The Massachusetts General Hospital Handbook of Internal Medicine.* Philadelphia: Lippincott Williams & Wilkins; 2000:6–3.

Tierney LM, McPhee SJ, Papadakis MA. *2006 Current Medical Diagnosis and Treatment.* 45th ed. New York: McGraw-Hill Companies, Inc; 2006: 937–939, 1431–1432, 1441.

Section II

Emergent Neurologic Conditions

Chapter 24

HEADACHE

Differential Diagnosis of Headache

Primary	Migraine
	Cluster
	Tension
Secondary	Subarachnoid hemorrhage
	Intracerebral hemorrhage
	Subdural/epidural hematoma
	Unruptured arteriovenous malformation
	Cerebral venous thrombosis
	Ischemic stroke/transient ischemic attack
	Cervicocephalic arterial dissection
	Arterial hypertension
	Meningitis
	Cerebral tumor/abscess
	Pseudotumor cerebri
	Postconcussive headache
	Acute glaucoma
	Trigeminal neuralgia
	Sinusitis
	Dental abscess
	Giant cell arthritis
	Bell palsy

Warning Signs of a Life-Threatening Headache

Clinical Features	Associated Features	Exam Findings
First headache	Nausea/vomiting	Opthalmologic findings
Sudden onset	Visual changes	Dysconjugate gaze
Severe intensity	Neck stiffness	Unequal pupils
Different/persistent headache	Fever and chills	Eye globe hard to palpation
Nocturnal worsening and/or awakening from sleep due to pain	Seizure	Conjunctival injection/lens clouding
	Hypertensive urgency/emergency	Visual field deficits
Age >50 years	Weight loss	Preretinal/retinal hemorrhage
Clouding of consciousness	Altered mental status	Papilledema
Recent head trauma		Head/neck
Onset with straining/change in position		Evidence of head/neck trauma (e.g., "raccoon eyes")

(Continued)

Clinical Features	Associated Features	Exam Findings
Onset with Valsalva maneuver		Temporal tenderness
		Lymphadenopathy
History of bleeding disorder		
Hypercoagulable state		
Cancer		
HIV/AIDS		Neurologic
		Mental status changes
		Focal neurologic signs
		Change in gait
		Presence of meningeal signs
		Evidence of bleeding diathesis
		Elevated blood pressure

Management

- Presence of signs and symptoms of a secondary headache require immediate evaluation aimed at identifying and managing the underlying cause. Consult medicine/neurology immediately.
- Immediate studies may entail the following:
  - CT head (e.g., acute bleed)
  - MRI head (e.g., subacute bleed, arteriovenous malformation, tumor)
  - Lumbar puncture
  - Complete blood cell count (CBC) with differential
  - Prothrombin Time, International Normalized Ratio (PT/INR) and Activated Partial Thromboplastin Time (aPTT)
  - Chemistry panel
- Other studies may include magnetic resonance angiography (MRA) and magnetic resonance venography (MRV) of the head, sinus CT scan, erythrocyte sedimentation rate, C-reactive protein, toxicology screen, hypercoagulable profile, renal/liver/thyroid function, urinalysis, chest x-ray, and EEG.

References

Biller J, ed. *Practical Neurology.* 2nd ed. Philadelphia: Lippincott Williams & Wilkins; 2002:244–258.

Green GB, Harris IS, Lin GA, et al., eds. *The Washington Manual of Medical Therapeutics.* 31st ed. Philadelphia: Lippincott Williams & Wilkins; 2004:549–550.

Manu P, Suarez RE, Barnett BJ, eds. *Handbook of Medicine in Psychiatry.* Arlington: American Psychiatric Publishing, Inc; 2006:161–170.

Tierney LM, McPhee SJ, Papadakis MA. *2006 Current Medical Diagnosis and Treatment.* 45th ed. New York: McGraw-Hill Companies, Inc; 2006:31–33.

Chapter 25

INTRACRANIAL HEMORRHAGE

Etiologies	Hypertension
	Bleeding disorders
	Monoamine oxidase inhibitor (MAOI) hypertensive reaction
	Amyloid angiopathy
	Vascular malformation (e.g., intracranial aneurysm, venous thrombosis)
	Primary/secondary brain tumors
	Hemorrhagic conversion of ischemic stroke
	Trauma
	Drug abuse (e.g., cocaine, amphetamines)
	High alcohol intake
Clinical features	Sudden, dramatic, and intense onset
	Severe headache
	Altered mental status
	Photo-/phonophobia
	Lethargy
	Meningeal signs (prominent with subarachnoid hemorrhage)
	Focal neurologic signs
	Nausea
	Vomiting
	Disequilibrium/dizziness (e.g., cerebellar hemorrhage)
	Seizures
Exam findings	Abnormal vital signs
	Altered level of consciousness
	Ocular signs
	• Papilledema
	• Visual field deficits
	• Conjugate gaze palsies
	Focal neurologic signs
	• Cranial nerve abnormalities
	• Lateralizing findings
	• Speech, motor, sensory deficits
	• Language, cognitive deficits
	Meningeal signs
	Evidence of craniocerebral trauma (e.g., "raccoon eyes")
	Cardiovascular findings (e.g., carotid bruits, arrhythmias)
	Evidence of bleeding diathesis
Management	Call 911/neurology immediately
	Prepare for transfer to intensive care unit
	ABC management
	IV access and slow infusion of normal saline solution

(*Continued*)

Frequent monitoring of vital signs, cardiac and neurologic status
Control of pain, nausea, vomiting, and seizures
Initial studies may include the following:
- Head CT
- Complete blood cell count with platelet count
- PT/INR and aPTT
- Chemistry panel
- Arterial blood gases if hypoxic
- Lateral cervical spine x-ray
- EKG
- Chest x-ray

References

Biller J, ed. *Practical Neurology.* 2nd ed. Philadelphia: Lippincott Williams & Wilkins; 2002:456–468, 793.

Green GB, Harris IS, Lin GA, et al., eds. *The Washington Manual of Medical Therapeutics.* 31st ed. Philadelphia: Lippincott Williams & Wilkins; 2004:541–542.

Tierney LM, McPhee SJ, Papadakis MA. *2006 Current Medical Diagnosis and Treatment.* 45th ed. New York: McGraw-Hill Companies, Inc; 2006:994–996.

Kaufman D. *Clinical Neurology for Psychiatrists.* Philadelphia: W.B. Saunders Company; 2001:276–277.

Chapter 26

MULTIPLE SCLEROSIS

Disease subtypes	Relapsing-remitting Primary progressive Secondary progressive
Clinical features	Peak age at disease onset: 20 to 45 years Episodic neurologic symptoms involving discrete areas separated by time Ophthalmic (common at onset) • Internuclear ophthalmoplegia (diplopia on lateral gaze) • Diplopia • Optic atrophy • Nystagmus • Retrobulbar neuritis Neurologic • Weakness/spastic paresis • Numbness • Tingling • Dysarthria • Ataxia • Incoordination • Scanning speech • Dysdiadochokinesia • Intention tremor • Sphincter disturbance (e.g., urinary urgency, hesitancy) Psychiatric manifestations • Suicidality (increased risk in male patients, early onset of disease, recent diagnosis) • Depression • Mania • Anxiety • Cognitive impairment (e.g., deficits in memory, attention, information-processing speed, learning, executive functions) • Euphoria • Emotional lability • Personality changes (e.g., increased irritability, apathy) • Rare psychosis
Diagnostic findings	MRI—multiple focal periventricular areas of demyelination Cerebrospinal fluid—elevated myelin basic protein, elevated immunoglobulin, presence of oligoclonal bands Abnormal visual/somatosensory evoked potentials
Management	Consult and coordinate care with neurology

(Continued)

Closely monitor and manage psychiatric illness, with careful attention for risk of suicidality

Treatment may include managing symptoms (e.g., pain, bladder dysfunction) and immune-modulating therapies including β-interferon and corticosteroids

References

Biller J. ed. *Practical Neurology.* 2nd ed. Philadelphia: Lippincott Williams & Wilkins; 2002:518–531.

Kaufman D. *Clinical Neurology for Psychiatrists.* Philadelphia: W.B. Saunders Company; 2001:369–385.

Tierney LM, McPhee SJ, Papadakis MA. *2006 Current Medical Diagnosis and Treatment.* 45th ed. New York: McGraw-Hill Companies, Inc; 2006:1014–1015.

Chapter 27

SEIZURE DISORDER

Subtypes	Partial • Simple partial • Complex partial Generalized • Absence (petit mal) • Atypical absence • Myoclonic • Tonic-clonic (grand mal) • Status epilepticus
Etiology	Trauma: head trauma, stroke, hemorrhage, anoxia, neurosurgery Mass lesions: arteriovenous malformations (AVM), tumor, cysticercosis Infection: encephalitis, meningitis, AIDS Medications: penicillin, quinolones, metronidazole, INH, tricyclic antidepressants, lithium, antipsychotics (e.g., clozapine), bupropion, cyclosporin, cocaine, PCP Drug-induced: alcohol, barbiturates, benzodiazepines, change in anticonvulsant drug levels Metabolic: hypo- or hyperglycemia, electrolyte disturbance, hypoxia, uremia, hepatic disease Psychiatric: nonepileptiform (of note, a significant percentage of patients have comorbid epileptiform and nonepileptiform seizures), somatoform disorders, anxiety disorders such as panic disorder, psychosis Degenerative disorders Vascular diseases
Clinical features	+/− aura and/or psychic symptoms (e.g., déjà vu) Automatism (e.g., lip smacking) Dystonic posturing Twitching Staring Deviation of head and eyes Impaired/loss of awareness (e.g., complex partial and generalized seizures) Myoclonic activity Tonic-clonic activity
Exam findings	Tongue/buccal injury due to biting Urine/bowel incontinence Postictal confusion Postictal sleepiness Postictal agitation Transient neurologic deficit Seizure-induced trauma +/− aspiration

(*Continued*)

Acute management	Consult neurology
	Maintain airway, breathing, circulation
	Position patient onto left side with head down
	Assess vital signs and pulse oximetry, obtain brief history and perform focused exam
	Establish IV access
	Check fingerstick glucose
	Immediate labs to consider include:
	Chemistry panel, Ca, Mg, PO4, complete blood cell count with differential, antiepileptic drug levels, hepatic function, toxicology screen, blood alcohol level
	Administer thiamine 100 mg IV before dextrose 50 ml 50% dextrose
	Consider lorazepam 0.1mg/kg at 1–2 mg/min IV; monitor closely for respiratory depression
	Status epilepticus—seizure >5 min or incomplete recovery of consciousness between 2 seizures
	Medical emergency—Call 911/institute code blue/call neurology immediately
	Lorazepam 0.1 mg/kg IV at 1–2 mg/min (max 4–6 mg in adults but increased risk of respiratory depression at higher doses); may repeat q5–10 min (max 80 mg/24 h)
	Diazepam 5–10 mg IV at 1–2 mg/min; may repeat q5–10 min (max 100 mg/24 h)
	Other anticonvulsants that may be used for seizure control include phenytoin, fosphenytoin
	Continuously reassess need for intubation

Nonepileptiform Seizure Disorder Features

Predisposing factors	Commonly seen in women, teenagers, children
	Childhood sexual abuse
	Comorbid psychiatric illness, including mood disorders, anxiety, psychosis, somatoform, personality disorders
	Primary and/or secondary gain (e.g., witnessed seizures)
	Presence of emotional triggers
Seizure activity	Gradual onset
	Atypical and asymmetric/asynchronous movements
	Lack of tonic phase
	Less stereotyped activity from seizure to seizure
	Duration lasting >5 min (longer than average epileptic seizure)
	Nonresponse to multiple anticonvulsants
	Pelvic thrusting
	Flailing/thrashing movements
	Rhythmic side-to-side movements
	Movements fluctuate in intensity and frequency due to fatigue
	Preserved consciousness
	Absence of seizure-related injury
	Absence of seizure activity during sleep
Postictal activity	Absence of postictal lethargy, fatigue
	Normal EEG
	Preserved recall of events during seizure activity

References

Biller J, ed. *Practical Neurology*. 2nd ed. Philadelphia: Lippincott Williams & Wilkins; 2002:66–75, 791–792.

Kaufman D. *Clinical Neurology for Psychiatrists*. Philadelphia: W.B. Saunders Company; 2001:226–256.

Manu P, Suarez RE, Barnett BJ, eds. *Handbook of Medicine in Psychiatry*. Arlington: American Psychiatric Publishing, Inc; 2006:181–193.

Yudofsky SC, Hales RE. *Essentials of Neuropsychiatry and Clinical Neurosciences*. Arlington: American Psychiatric Publishing, Inc; 2004:297–298.

Chapter 28

STROKE LOCALIZATION

Internal carotid artery	May present with some or all of the features of infarctions involving the anterior cerebral, middle cerebral, and ophthalmic arteries
Anterior cerebral artery	Contralateral lower extremity paresis and/or sensory loss With bilateral infarcts, the following can be seen: Bilateral lower extremity motor impairment, frontal release signs, mutism, apathy, pseudobulbar palsy
Middle cerebral artery	Aphasia (dominant) Contralateral neglect/dressing difficulty (nondominant) Contralateral homonymous hemianopsia Contralateral hemiparesis/hemisensory loss
Posterior cerebral artery	Alexia without agraphia Contralateral homonymous hemianopsia Midbrain involvement: vertical gaze palsy, 3rd nerve palsy with contralateral hemiplegia (Weber syndrome) Thalamic involvement: amnesia, contralateral sensory disturbance, occasional tremor
Vertebral artery	Lateral medullary involvement (Wallenberg syndrome): ipsilateral ataxia, vertigo, nystagmus, ipsilateral Horner syndrome (droopy lid and small pupil), ipsilateral pharyngeal and laryngeal paralysis (leading to hoarseness), ipsilateral sensory loss of face/contralateral sensory loss of body (pain/temperature) Cerebellar involvement: ipsilateral limb ataxia, dysmetria, dysarthria, vertigo, nausea, nystagmus
Basilar artery	Midbrain involvement: complete or partial 3rd nerve palsy, contralateral motor involvement Pontine involvement: ipsilateral 6th nerve paresis, contralateral motor involvement Lateral medullary involvement: ipsilateral limb ataxia, palatal paresis, Horner syndrome Total occlusion → coma, locked-in syndrome

References

Kaufman D. *Clinical Neurology for Psychiatrists*. Philadelphia: W.B. Saunders Company; 2001:268–283.

Lindsay KW, Bone I. *Neurology and Neurosurgery Illustrated*. London: Churchill Livingstone; 1999:243–253.

Stern TA, Herman JB. *Massachusetts General Hospital Psychiatry Update and Board Preparation*. 2nd ed. New York: McGraw-Hill; 2000:310–311.

Chapter 29

TRANSIENT ISCHEMIC ATTACK/STROKE

Clinical features	Altered mental status
	Visual changes (e.g., diplopia/vision loss)
	Dysphagia
	Facial droop
	Aphasia, dysarthria, word-finding
	Focal motor impairment
	Focal sensory impairment
	Dizziness/vertigo
	Ataxia
	Loss of fine motor skills
	Frontal release signs
	Loss of executive function
Exam findings	Altered mental status
	Neurologic findings—lateralizing signs
	• Neglect
	• Aphasia
	• Apraxia
	• Visual field deficits
	• Ocular palsies
	• Facial weakness
	• Hemiparesis
	• Hemisensory disturbance
	• Hemiataxia
	Meningeal signs
	Cardiovascular findings
	• Arrhythmia (e.g., atrial fibrillation, mitral/atrial stenosis)
	• Murmurs
	Evidence of embolic disease
Management	Consult neurology immediately
	Prepare patient for transfer to intensive care unit
	Assess airway, breathing, and circulation
	Vital signs to evaluate for hemodynamic instability, oxygen saturation, fever, respiratory drive
	NPO except medications
	Ensure administration of oxygen and placement of intravenous fluid access
	Aspiration precautions
	Medications
	Do not administer aspirin, heparin, or other blood thinners until intracranial bleed is ruled out
	Consider aspirin 160–325 mg/d
	Do not treat hypertension

(Continued)

Diagnostic studies may include the following:
- Arterial blood gases if hypoxic
- 12-lead EKG
- Head CT non-contrast or MRI stroke protocol
- Complete blood cell count with differential
- Chemistry panel
- Fingerstick glucose
- Blood cultures if fever present
- PT/INR and aPTT
- Chest x-ray if suspect lung or heart disease
- Toxicology screen

References

Biller J, ed. *Practical Neurology.* 2nd ed. Philadelphia: Lippincott Williams & Wilkins; 2002:439–455.

Green GB, Harris IS, Lin GA, et al., eds. *The Washington Manual of Medical Therapeutics.* 31st ed. Philadelphia: Lippincott Williams & Wilkins; 2004:539–541.

Kaufman D. *Clinical Neurology for Psychiatrists.* Philadelphia: W.B. Saunders Company; 2001:268–283.

Rosen H. *The Consult Manual of Internal Medicine.* Med Consult Publishing Inc; 2006:768–775.

Section III

Neuropsychiatry

Chapter 30

DELIRIUM

Differential Diagnosis of Delirium

	Delirium	Dementia	Depression	Schizophrenia
Onset	Acute	Often insidious	Variable	Variable
Course	Fluctuating	Often progressive	Diurnal variation	Variable
Reversibility	Usually	Not usually	Usually, but can be recurrent	No
Level of consciousness	Impaired	Clear until late stages	Usually unimpaired	Not impaired, but perplexity seen in acute illness
Attention/memory	Poor memory and attention	Poor memory without marked inattention	Poor attention, memory intact	Poor attention, memory intact
Hallucinations	Usually vivid visual and tactile; but any modality possible	Visual or auditory	Usually auditory	Usually auditory
Delusions	Fleeting, fragmented, usually persecutory with local context (e.g., hospital is a prison)	Paranoid, often fixed	Complex and mood congruent	Frequent, complex, systematized, often paranoid

Modified from Hales RE, Yudofsky SC, eds. *Essentials of Neuropsychiatry and Clinical Neurosciences.* Washington, DC: American Psychiatric Publishing, Inc; 2004:144, with permission.

Clinical Features

- Sleep-wake disturbance.
- Psychosis: perceptual disturbance (especially visual hallucinations), delusions, disorganized thought process.
- Abnormalities of mood and affect: altered or labile, usually incongruent with mood.

- Motor: hyperactive, hypoactive, mixed.
- Cognition: impairments in attention, memory, and executive function.
- Fluctuating course.

Evaluation of Delirium

- Complete history: chart review, collateral data, vulnerabilities (pre-existing cognitive/sensory impairment, central nervous system disorders), current medical illness.
- Medication review: include temporal sequence correlated with medication changes. Pay particular attention to recently administered medications, including drug–drug interactions, herbal, illicit, prescription, and over-the-counter drugs. Common medications precipitating delirium include opiates, anticholinergics/antihistamines, sedative-hypnotics, steroids, H2-blockers, antibiotics, cardiac drugs, and antineoplastic agents.
- Vital signs, including orthostatics and oxygen saturation.
- Examination: physical, neurologic, psychiatric.
- Cognitive evaluation:
  - Mini-Mental State Exam (MMSE). The most sensitive items test orientation, attention/concentration (e.g., serial 7s), and memory. Serial MMSEs may be helpful in following the course of the delirium.
  - Clock draw, Trails B (tests concentration, visual scanning, and cognitive flexibility).
  - Frontal release signs.
  - Rating scales—the Delirium Rating scale, Confusion Assessment Method, Memorial Delirium Assessment scale, Delirium Symptom Interview.
- Labs as clinically appropriate, including complete blood cell count (CBC) with differential, chemistry panel, including Ca, Mg, PO4, tests of hepatic function, ammonia, toxicology screen, urinalysis, arterial blood gases, B12, folate, medication serum levels (digoxin, dilantin, phenobarbital, coumadin, theophylline). Other tests to consider may be blood cultures, HIV, antinuclear antibodies (ANA), cerebrospinal fluid (CSF) studies, rapid plasma reagin (RPR)/Venereal Disease Research Laboratory test (VDRL).
- Studies: chest x-ray, EKG, brain imaging, EEG (diffuse slowing).

Pharmacotherapy*

Agent	Dosage	Special Considerations
Haloperidol	2–10 mg p.o./IM/IV BID and q4h prn agitation In elderly, administer starting dose at 25%–50% of adult doses.	QTc** >450 msec or to greater than 25% over baseline EKG predicts development of torsades de pointes

(Continued)

Agent	Dosage	Special Considerations
	Repeat or double dose in 30–60 min until patient is calm (check QTc before repeating dose). If no response with 2 escalating doses, consider adding benzodiazepine. Once patient is calm, add total mg of Haldol and administer same amount orally divided BID-TID over the next 24 h. Taper by 50% q24h assuming patient remains calm.	and may warrant dose reduction or discontinuation. Consult cardiology and transfer patient to telemetry unit. Monitor for excess sedation and extrapyramidal symptoms.
Olanzapine	2.5–10 mg p.o./IM BID with 2.5–5 mg q8 prn agitation (max 20 mg/24 h).	For IM administration, wait 2–4 h between doses. Monitor for excess sedation and orthostatic hypotension. Elderly patients with dementia-related psychosis treated with atypical antipsychotic drugs are at an increased risk of death compared to placebo.
Risperidone	0.5–4 mg/d divided BID-TID.	Elderly patients with dementia-related psychosis treated with atypical antipsychotic drugs are at an increased risk of death compared to placebo. Increased risk of extrapyramidal symptoms compared with other atypical antipsychotics.
Quetiapine	25–200 mg/d divided BID-QID and 6.25–25 mg p.o. q4 prn agitation (max 400 mg/24 h).	Monitor for excess sedation and orthostatic hypotension. May be agent of choice when indicated for use with comorbid movement disorders characterized by parkinsonian features.

*This table includes medications not FDA approved for delirium.
**Risk factors for QTc include hypokalemia, hypomagnesemia, bradycardia, congenital long-QT syndrome, preexisting cardiac disease, drug–drug interactions.

Risk Factors for Delirium and Intervention Protocols

Targeted Risk Factor and Eligible Patients	Standardized Intervention Protocols
Cognitive impairment: All patients, protocol once daily; patients with baseline MMSE score of <20 and orientation score of <8, protocol 3× daily.	Orientation protocol: board with names of care-team members and day's schedule; communication to reorient to surroundings. Therapeutic activities protocol: cognitively stimulating activities 3× daily (e.g., discussion of current events, structured reminiscence, word games).
Sleep deprivation: All patients, need for protocol assessed once daily.	Nonpharmacological sleep protocol: at bedtime, warm drink (milk or herbal tea), relaxation tapes or music, and back massage. Sleep-enhancement protocol: unitwide noise-reduction strategies (e.g., silent pill crushers, vibrating beepers, and quiet hallways) and schedule adjustments to allow sleep (e.g., rescheduling of medications and procedures).
Immobility: All patients, ambulation whenever possible, and range-of-motion exercises when patient is chronically nonambulatory, bed- or wheelchair-bound, or immobilized (e.g., because of an extremity fracture or deep venous thrombosis), or has been prescribed bed rest.	Early mobilization protocol: ambulation or active range-of-motion exercises 3× daily; minimal use of immobilizing equipment (e.g., bladder catheters, physical restraints).
Visual impairment: Patients with <20/70 visual acuity on binocular near-vision testing.	Vision protocol: visual aids (e.g., glasses or magnifying lenses) and adaptive equipment (e.g., large illuminated telephone keypads, large-print books, fluorescent tape on call bell), with daily reinforcement of their use.
Hearing impairment: Patients with <7 of 12 whispers on Whisper Test.	Hearing protocol: portable amplifying devices, earwax disimpaction, and special communication techniques, with daily reinforcement of these adaptations.
Dehydration: Patients with ratio of blood urea nitrogen to creatinine of >17, screened for protocol by geriatric nurse-specialist.	Dehydration protocol: early recognition of dehydration and volume repletion (e.g., encouragement of oral intake fluids).

Reprinted from Hales RE, Yudofsky SC, eds. *The American Psychiatric Publishing Textbook of Clinical Psychiatry.* 4th ed. Washington, DC: American Psychiatric Publishing, Inc; 2003:273, with permission.

Adapted with permission from Inouye SK, Bogardus ST, Jr, Charpentier PA, et al. A multicomponent intervention to prevent delirium in hospitalized older patients. *New England Journal of Medicine.* 1999; 340:669–676. Copyright © 1999 Massachusetts Medical Society All rights reserved.

References

Hales RE, Yudofsky SC, eds. *Essentials of Neuropsychiatry and Clinical Neurosciences.* Washington, DC: American Psychiatric Publishing, Inc; 2004:141–175.

Hales RE, Yudofsky SC, eds. *The American Psychiatric Publishing Textbook of Clinical Psychiatry.* 4th ed. Washington, DC: American Psychiatric Publishing, Inc; 2003:259–274.

Chapter 31

DEMENTIA

Epidemiology

- Average age from diagnosis to death is 3 to 10 years.
- Risk increases exponentially with age from 1% under age 65 to 25%–50% over age 85.

Characteristics of Cortical and Subcortical Dementias*

Characteristics	Cortical Dementia	Subcortical
Attention	Decreased	Decreased
Memory	Prominent memory impairment Recognition deficits >recall	Retrieval and recall deficits >recognition Less severe intellectual and memory dysfunction
Language	Prominent deficits with aphasia and agnosia	Decreased verbal fluency without anomia Dysarthria may be present
Executive function	Varies with course	Poor and disproportionately affected
Cognition	Impaired judgment, abstraction, and calculation	Impaired problem solving and decision making
Emotion	Absent early in disease Tendency to minimize deficits Psychosis/agitation later in course	Apathy Prominent affective changes with depressed mood/affective lability
Motivation	Alert, attentive, ambulatory	Decreased with bradyphrenia (slowed mental processing)
Motor abnormalities	Lack prominent signs Preserved motor function, gait, and posture Apraxia	Prominent with gait abnormalities Tremor, tics, dystonia, extrapyramidal symptoms may be present
Visuospatial skills	Present	Later in disease
Examples	Alzheimer type Frontotemporal Creutzfeldt–Jakob disease	Dementias due to HIV, Parkinson disease, Huntington disease, multiple sclerosis

*Of note, the dichotomies outlined above are not absolute. Features may often overlap depending on increasing severity and location of illness (e.g., vascular and Lewy body dementias demonstrate combined features).

Distinguishing Features of Dementia of the Alzheimer Type (DAT) and Frontotemporal Dementia

Features	Dementia of the Alzheimer Type	Frontotemporal Dementia
Course	Insidious onset and steady progression	Earlier age (<65) Insidious onset and slow progression
Presenting symptoms	Memory loss with poor insight Impaired functioning in independent activities such as driving to unfamiliar places and financial management	Personality changes Social and personal disinhibition Affective blunting Loss of insight
Cognitive deficits	Memory impairment Language disturbance Impaired executive functioning Apraxia and agnosia	Intact visuospatial skills Severe impairment in executive functions Progressive expressive aphasia and mutism later in course
Mood/personality disturbances	**Mood** Depression common, especially in mild cases Anxiety Affective lability Agitation with worsening of illness **Personality** Disinhibition common Apathy and agitation increase as illness progresses	**Mood** Prominent depression Suicidality Anxiety **Personality** Severe apathy and disinhibition (e.g., sexually and aggressive)
Psychotic/behavioral disturbances	**Psychosis** Delusions: persecutory, theft themes common Visual hallucinations common **Behavioral** Increasing agitation (e.g., wandering, pacing) as disease progresses Verbal and physical aggression often accompanies psychosis	**Psychosis** Bizarre delusions **Behavioral** Poor social and interpersonal regulation and awareness Stereotyped and impulsive behavior Severe compulsions (e.g., hyperorality) Somatic preoccupation
Motor abnormalities	Not prominent early in disease	Frontal lobe release reflexes early in course

(*Continued*)

Features	Dementia of the Alzheimer Type	Frontotemporal Dementia
	Visuospatial difficulties (e.g., constructional apraxia)	Akinesia/bradykinesia, ataxia, perseveration of movements, rigidity, and tremor late in course
Neuropathology	Neuritic plaques consisting of beta-amyloid protein deposits Neurofibrillary tangles consisting of hyperphosphorylated tau Loss of neurons in the nucleus basalis of Meynert	Frontal and anterior temporal lobe atrophy Abnormal function of the cytoskeletal protein tau Pick disease: presence of massed argentophilic inclusion-containing neurons (Pick's bodies)
Special considerations	Typical decline in MMSE scores in DAT is 2–4 points per year Risk factors include family history, limited cognitive reserve, increased age, female, smoking, never married, Down syndrome, apolipoprotein E (APOE) e4 allele, history of head trauma Higher educational attainment/increased cognitive reserve is protective	May be misdiagnosed as substance use, hypomania, personality disorders, and/or schizophrenia

Subcortical Dementias

Dementia due to HIV/AIDS
- Refer to Chapter 36 on HIV/AIDS.

Dementia due to Parkinson disease
- Refer to Chapter 33 on Parkinson disease.

Dementia due to Huntington disease
- Refer to Chapter 32 on Huntington disease.

Dementia due to multiple sclerosis
- Refer to Chapter 26 on multiple sclerosis.

Dementia with Cortical and Subcortical Cardinal Features

Vascular Dementia (VaD)

- Abrupt onset, stepwise progression, with relative stability of cognitive status between vascular insults.

- Focal neurologic signs and symptoms with patchy cognitive deficits.
- Presence of cardiovascular disease.
- Personality changes, depression, affective instability, and somatic preoccupation common.
- Post-stroke dementia
  - Often preceded by stroke in the dominant hemisphere.
  - Risk factors include presence of comorbid medical illness (e.g., diabetes mellitus), decreased cognitive reserve, and demographics such as advanced age and non-white race.
  - Major depression common and typically associated with dominant/left hemispheric stroke.
  - Treatment with selective serotonin reuptake inhibitors (SSRIs) may result in decreased long-term mortality rates possibly secondary to improved compliance with post-stroke treatment regimens and intrinsic antiplatelet effects.

Dementia with Lewy Bodies (LBD)

- Fluctuating mental status, extrapyramidal symptoms, visual hallucinations, and systematized delusions.
- Deficits in attention, visuospatial skills, and executive function.
- Psychosis and agitation are initially managed with acetylcholinesterase inhibitors.
- Due to extreme sensitivity to neuroleptic agents (e.g., exacerbation of extrapyramidal symptoms, further cognitive decline), consider augmentation with newer atypical antipsychotics, such as quetiapine. Avoid clozapine due to potential worsening of fall risk in these patients (due to anticholinergic effects).

Differential Diagnosis of Cognitive Decline

- Central nervous system disorders
  - Vascular
  - Mass lesions
  - Infections (e.g., meningitis, HIV/AIDS, neurosyphilis)
  - Head trauma
  - Autoimmune
- Psychiatric illness
  - Major depression (pseudodementia)
  - Substance intoxication or withdrawal
  - Delirium
  - Psychotic disorders
- Systemic illness
  - Hepatic failure
  - Renal failure
- Nutritional deficiencies
  - Thiamine
  - Niacin
  - Vitamin B_{12}
- Metabolic/endocrine disorders
  - Hypothyroidism

- Hypercalcemia
- Hypoglycemia
- Adrenal
- Medications
  - Steroids
  - Pain medications
  - Anticholinergic agents
  - Heavy metals

Comprehensive Dementia Workup

- Physical exam including thorough neurologic exam
- Vital signs
- Mental status exam
- Mini-Mental State Exam (MMSE)
- Review of medications and drug levels
- Blood and urine screens for alcohol, drugs, and heavy metals
- Physiologic workup
  - Complete blood count with differential
  - Electrolytes, glucose, Ca^{2+}, Mg^{2+}, PO_4^{2-}
  - Liver and renal function tests
  - Urinalysis and toxicology screen
  - TSH
  - Rapid plasma regain (RPR) and fluorescent treponemal antibody absorption test (FTA-ABS)
  - Serum B_{12} and folate
  - Erythrocyte sedimentation rate (ESR)
  - HIV status in high-risk groups
  - If indicated by history and physical, urine corticosteroids, rheumatoid screen (antinuclear antibodies [ANA], C3/C4, anti-ds DNA), arterial blood gases, urine porphobilinogens
- Chest x-ray
- EKG
- Neurologic workup if indicated
  - CT or MRI head scan
  - Single photon emission CT (SPECT)
  - Lumbar puncture
  - EEG

Management
Stages of Dementia

Stage of Impairment	Features	Likely Symptoms
Normal aging	Annoying but not disabling problems, such as forgetting names and minor difficulties in recalling detailed events	Subjective memory complaints

(Continued)

Stage of Impairment	Features	Likely Symptoms
Mild cognitive impairment (MCI)	Problem is not disabling, but with noticeable change in memory noted by informants	Subjective memory complaints Memory performance 1.5 standard deviations below age-matched peers
Mild	Difficulties limited to complex tasks such as balancing a checkbook	Depression Awareness of & frustration with deficits
Moderate	Difficulty completing simple household tasks	Depression Development of psychotic symptoms such as paranoia
Severe	Requires assistance with basic activities of daily living such as personal hygiene	Psychosis Agitation
Profound	Terminal and totally dependent	Bedbound with significant motor deficits Feeding difficulties Incontinence

Adapted from American Psychiatric Association, Treating Alzheimer's disease and other dementias of late life. In: *Quick Reference to the American Psychiatric Association Practice Guidelines for the Treatment of Psychiatric Disorders, Compendium 2006*. American Psychiatric Association Steering Committee on Practice Guidelines, p. 38; and Spar JE, La Rue A. *Concise Guide to Geriatric Psychiatry.* 3rd ed. Washington, DC: American Psychiatric Publishing, Inc; 2002:194.

Management of Dementia

Pharmacotherapy General Considerations

- Start with low doses and titrate gradually due to decreased renal clearance and slowed hepatic metabolism in the elderly.
- The elderly are more sensitive to potential side effects of medications, including development of delirium, falls secondary to orthostatic hypotension and sedation, as well as extrapyramidal symptoms.
- Be cognizant of comorbid medical conditions, such as cardiovascular disease and diabetes mellitus.
- Avoid polypharmacy.
- Coordinate care with primary care provider and keep apprised of any new treatment decisions.

Cognitive Enhancers

ACETYLCHOLINESTERASE INHIBITORS

- Donepezil 5 mg/day (maximum 10 mg/day). Major side effects include gastrointestinal (GI) upset, fatigue, anorexia, bradycardia, syncope.
- Rivastigmine 1.5 mg twice/day (maximum 6 mg twice/day). Cholinesterase inhibitor with effects on both acetylcholinesterase

and butyrylcholinesterase with a theoretical benefit in advanced dementia of the Alzheimer type. May be associated with increased GI side effects compared to donepezil.
- Galantamine 4 mg twice/day (maximum 12 mg twice/day). Metabolized by cytochrome p450 2D6/3A4 and clearance may be decreased by inhibitors of these enzymes.

N-Methyl-D-Aspartic Acid (NMDA) Antagonists

- Memantine 5 mg/day (maximum 10 mg twice/day). Typically used for augmentation of moderate to severe Alzheimer disease. Major side effects include agitation, hallucinations, dizziness, and constipation. Avoid coadministration with other NMDA antagonists (e.g., dextromethorphan) due to risk of psychosis.

Antidepressants

- SSRIs are often the preferred class of antidepressants in dementia patients.
- Caution with use of paroxetine due to significant anticholinergic activity.
- SSRIs may also be useful in managing sexual disinhibition, poor impulse control, agitation, and apathy.
- Other antidepressants may be helpful by virtue of their side-effect profile (e.g., mirtazapine in elderly with anorexia and insomnia).

Anticonvulsants

- May be indicated for agitation, aggression, and mood lability.
- Caution with agents associated with increased risk of delirium and cognitive impairment (e.g., lithium and beta-blockers).

Antipsychotics

- Indicated for psychosis, delirium, and agitation.
- Elderly patients with dementia-related psychosis treated with atypical antipsychotic drugs are at an increased risk of death compared to placebo.
- Caution in use with risk factors or previous history of cerebral vascular incidents.
- Careful selection of antipsychotic agent with due consideration of comorbid medical illnesses and side-effect profile.
- Follow-up monitoring should include physical health and laboratory monitoring, as well as examination for medication-induced movement disorders with the Assessment of Involuntary Movements scale.

Anxiolytics

- Use benzodiazepines with extreme caution due to the high risk of further cognitive impairment, excessive sedation, delirium, and falls.

Psychostimulants

- May be effective in improving apathy with smaller effects on mood and cognition.
- Methylphenidate 2.5–5 mg/day is a recommended starting dose.

Miscellaneous

- NSAIDs may delay disease progression in dementia through anti-inflammatory mechanisms.
- Factors such as diet (e.g., dietary intake of fish), vitamins C and E, alpha-tocopherol, and physical/cognitive fitness may lower risk of dementia of the Alzheimer type.

Environmental and Behavioral Management

- The patient should always carry and/or wear identification.
- Safety considerations
  - Alter environment (e.g., remove loose rugs).
  - Remove weapons from the home or secure in a locked cabinet.
  - Provide adequate lighting, including night-light.
  - Organize home to simplify routines, including having emergency phone numbers easily accessible.
- Consider respite care to decrease burden on primary caregivers, to include in-home caregivers, adult day care centers/senior centers, and supportive psychotherapy for caregivers.

Legal Aspects of Management

- Advise the patient early in the course of illness to complete medicolegal documents (e.g., advance directives).
- Document above discussion, including any wishes communicated by the patient.
- Driving: Be aware of disclosure laws regarding notification of dementia diagnosis to state motor vehicle departments. Coordinate decision with primary care provider and take into consideration other sensory and motor deficits.
- Address any signs of neglect or abuse.

Outpatient Management

- Early discussion of diagnosis, prognosis, and management with frequent clinical follow-ups.
- Continuously assess whether the patient can live safely at home.
- Indications for 24-h supervision include escalating violence, inability to perform activities of daily living, dangerous behaviors (e.g., leaving stove on), and wandering away from home.
- Assess for caregiver burden during each visit.
- Continuously monitor patient's potential for suicide and violence.
- Simplify patient's medication regimen, including avoiding polypharmacy, minimizing orthostatic hypotension and delirium risk, and preventing accidental overdose.

Resources

The 36-Hour Day: A Family Guide to Caring for Persons with Alzheimer's Disease, Related Dementing Illnesses, and Memory Loss in Later Life (Warner Books, 1981).

Alzheimer's Association (1-800-621-0379); www.alz.org

The Alzheimer's Association can facilitate patient enrollment in the Safe Return Program, a nationwide program that assists in the identification and return of dementia patients who wander.

References

Blazer DG, Steffens DC, Busse EW, eds. *The American Psychiatric Publishing Textbook of Geriatric Psychiatry.* 3rd ed. Washington, DC: American Psychiatric Publishing, Inc; 2004:209–221.

Hales RE, Yudofsky SC, eds. *The American Psychiatric Publishing Textbook of Clinical Psychiatry.* 4th ed. Washington, DC: American Psychiatric Publishing, Inc; 2003:274–293.

Kaufman D. *Clinical Neurology for Psychiatrists.* Philadelphia: W.B. Saunders Company; 2001:132–143.

Mace NJ, Rabins PV. *The 36-Hour Day: A Family Guide to Caring for Persons with Alzheimer's Disease, Related Dementing Illnesses, and Memory Loss in Later Life.* New York: Warner Books; 1981.

Quick Reference to the American Psychiatric Association Practice Guidelines for the Treatment of Psychiatric Disorders, Compendium 2006. Arlington, VA: American Psychiatric Association; 32–47.

Sadock BJ, Sadock VA. *Kaplan & Sadock's Synopsis of Psychiatry: Behavioral Sciences/Clinical Psychiatry.* 9th ed. Philadelphia, PA: Lippincott Williams & Wilkins; 2003:329–338.

Spar JE, La Rue A. *Concise Guide to Geriatric Psychiatry.* 3rd ed. Washington, DC: American Psychiatric Publishing, Inc; 2002:153–190, 197–220.

Wendling P. Methylphenidate may improve apathy associated with dementia. *Clin Psychiatr News.* 2006;34:(8):43.

Yudofsky SC, Hales RE. *Essentials of Neuropsychiatry and Clinical Neurosciences.* Washington DC: American Psychiatric Publishing, Inc; 2004:422–432.

Chapter 32

HUNTINGTON DISEASE

Epidemiology	Onset between 30 and 50 years of age Average life expectancy ~15 years Male = female
Cardinal features	Triad of dyskinesia, dementia, and behavioral abnormalities Autosomal dominant with complete penetrance Chromosome 4 Unstable CAG trinucleotide repeat
Clinical features	**Dyskinesia** Chorea Dysarthria Dystonia Rigidity **Dementia** Subcortical type Impaired cognitive flexibility Psychomotor difficulties Difficulties with complex tasks Language and memory intact until late in disease **Behavioral abnormalities** Often herald onset of illness Irritability/aggression common Depression (30%–50%)—may precede onset of motor abnormalities by several years Increased suicidality and suicide rate (up to 25% attempt suicide at least once) Mania/hypomania Anxiety Obsessive compulsive disorders Psychosis Sexual disorders
Diagnostic considerations	DNA testing is definitive and is available for patients and potential carriers, including a fetus Central nervous system imaging demonstrates atrophy of the caudate and putamen Functional imaging reveals decreased metabolism in the caudate nucleus
Management considerations	Progressive illness with no cure Symptom management is the mainstay of treatment **Dyskinesia** Dopamine antagonists (e.g., antipsychotics) may reduce the severity of the dyskinesia and behavioral abnormalities Consider antipsychotics with decreased inherent risk for extrapyramidal symptoms and tardive dyskinesia

(Continued)

Dementia
　No specific treatments available for management of cognitive impairment

Behavioral abnormalities

Aggression
- Management of aggression should target underlying cause:
  　Antipsychotics for aggression secondary to psychosis
  　Antidepressants for depression-related suicidality
  　Mood stabilizers for mania-related agitation
  　Propranolol for general aggression and irritability

Depression
　Selective serotonin reuptake inhibitors (SSRIs) are the mainstay of treatment
　Consider mirtazapine in patients with anorexia and insomnia
　Careful monitoring of suicide risk, including access to weapons

Mania/hypomania
- Management may entail use of mood stabilizers (e.g., lithium, valproic acid, carbamazepine) and benzodiazepines

Psychosis
- Consider antipsychotics with decreased inherent risk for extrapyramidal symptoms and tardive dyskinesia

References

Biller J, ed. *Practical Neurology.* 2nd ed. Philadelphia: Lippincott Williams & Wilkins; 2002:543–544.

Blazer DG, Steffens DC, Busse EW, eds. *The American Psychiatric Publishing Textbook of Geriatric Psychiatry.* 3rd ed. Washington, DC: American Psychiatric Publishing, Inc; 2004:193–197.

Kaufman D. *Clinical Neurology for Psychiatrists.* Philadelphia: W.B. Saunders Company; 2001:458–465.

Tierney LM, McPhee SJ, Papadakis MA. *2006 Current Medical Diagnosis and Treatment.* 45th ed. New York: McGraw-Hill Companies, Inc; 2006:1010–1011.

Yudofsky SC, Hales RE. *Essentials of Neuropsychiatry and Clinical Neurosciences.* Washington, DC: American Psychiatric Publishing, Inc; 2004:430–432.

Chapter 33

PARKINSON DISEASE

Epidemiology	Onset between 45 and 65 years of age
	Approximately equal sex and ethnic distribution
	Risk factors for development of dementia include increased age, greater severity of neurologic symptoms, and presence of APOE e2 allele
Cardinal features of parkinsonian syndrome	4–6 Hz resting tremor
	Rigidity
	Bradykinesia
	Postural instability
Clinical features	**Motor**
	General
	Unilateral onset
	Persistent asymmetry affecting side of onset most
	Excellent initial response (70%–100%) to levodopa
	Bradykinesia
	Masked facies
	Decreased blinking
	Hypophonic speech
	Prolonged response latency
	Slowed festinating gait with decreased arm swing
	Micrographia
	Rigidity
	Trunk & limb muscles
	Cogwheeling
	Tremor
	Resting
	Typically, pill-rolling
	Cognitive
	Characterized by dementia of the subcortical type (please refer to Chapter 31)
	Antiparkinsonian medications frequently exacerbate cognitive impairment
	Treatment of comorbid mood disorders may improve cognition
	Psychiatric
	Mood
	~50% depression
	Prominent features include anxiety and increased suicidality
	Anxiety
	Typically Generalized Anxiety Disorder
	Panic disorder, obsessive compulsive disorders, and discrete phobias have also been observed
	Psychosis
	Characterized by visual hallucinations, delusions, confusion
	Fluctuates during day, worse in evening

(Continued)

	Often associated with longstanding parkinsonian illness, high doses of antiparkinson medications, and dementia
	Sleep disturbances
	Increased time to sleep onset with multiple awakenings
	Vivid, disconcerting dreams
Diagnosis	Clinical diagnosis strongly suggested by history and physical exam
	Central nervous system imaging, particularly MRI, is indicated in the presence of remarkably unilateral neurologic findings to rule out mass lesion or in the event of atypical neurologic findings
	MRI shows reductions in the size of substantia nigra in advanced cases of Parkinson disease
Management	**General considerations**
	Coordinate care with neurologists and other specialists including physical therapy, dietician, social workers
	Psychoeducation for patient, family, caregivers
	Assessment of functional limitations, including activities of daily living, gait disturbance, fall risk
	Attention to caregiver burden
	Hallucinations and delusions typically occur at night and are the chief reason families place patients in nursing homes
	Treatment of movement disorder
	Therapy often entails slowing the progression of the disease with neuroprotective agents (e.g., selegiline) followed by symptomatic treatment with agents such as dopamine agonists and anticholinergics
	Neuroprotective agents such as selegiline can slow the progression of the disorder and thus defer the need for dopaminergic therapy
	Despite levodopa therapy, parkinsonian motor symptoms reemerge after 5–10 years
	For patients unable to tolerate levodopa, amantadine and dopamine receptor agonists are useful adjuncts in the therapy of Parkinson disease
	Surgical procedures include stereotactic ventral pallidotomy, deep brain stimulation, or transplantation
	Treatment of comorbid psychiatric symptoms
	When possible, simplify/optimize medication regimens
	Rule out underlying metabolic and infectious causes for perceptual and mood disturbances
	Psychotic symptoms are common adverse effects of antiparkinsonism medications
	Consider discontinuation of antiparkinsonism medications in the following order: anticholinergics > amantadine > selegiline > dopaminergic agents
	Persistent psychotic symptoms warrant use of antipsychotic agents
	Clozapine and quetiapine at low doses are preferred agents due to decreased inherent risk of extrapyramidal symptoms

(Continued)

Mood and anxiety symptoms may respond to dopaminergic agent dose reductions

Rule out parkinsonian drug-associated psychiatric symptoms

Visual hallucinations, typically characterized by human or animal figures, usually at night

Persecutory delusions

Elevated mood

Anxiety

Increased sexual interest

Management includes discontinuation of anticholinergic medications, dosage adjustment of antiparkinsonian medications, and/or addition of neuroleptic agents for persistent psychotic symptoms (consider Clozaril or Seroquel to minimize extrapyramidal symptoms)

References

Biller J, ed. *Practical Neurology.* 2nd ed. Philadelphia: Lippincott Williams & Wilkins; 2002:346–349, 532–542.

Kaufman D. *Clinical Neurology for Psychiatrists.* Philadelphia: W.B. Saunders Company; 2001:445–457.

Yudofsky SC, Hales RE. *Essentials of Neuropsychiatry and Clinical Neurosciences.* Washington, DC: American Psychiatric Publishing, Inc; 2004:432–435.

Chapter 34

SLEEP DISORDERS

Sleep Disorders and Psychiatric Illness

Depression	Insomnia: present in the majority of patients with major depression
	Generalized sleep disturbance:
	  Increased time to sleep onset
	  Increased nighttime awakenings
	  Early morning awakenings
	Sleep architecture findings:
	  Decreased slow-wave sleep
	  Decreased rapid eye movement (REM) latency
	Medication effects:
	  Selective serotonin reuptake inhibitors (SSRIs) may cause insomnia—increased REM latency, decreased REM duration, sleep fragmentation, increased awakenings, increased dreaming/nightmares/sexual dreams/obsessions (with fluoxetine)
	  Trazodone—increased sleep onset, improved sleep quality, increased REM latency, decreased REM duration, increased slow-wave sleep
	  Bupropion—decreased REM latency, increased REM sleep, decreased sleep continuity and slow-wave sleep, vivid dreams/nightmares

Mania and hypomania	Increased time to sleep onset Reduced slow-wave sleep
Schizophrenia	Decreased sleep continuity Increased time to sleep onset Sleep fragmentation with multiple arousals Decreased slow-wave sleep
Anxiety	Decreased sleep continuity Increased time to sleep onset Increased sleep fragmentation No change in REM latency or percentage of REM sleep
Substance-related (alcohol)	Decreased REM sleep the first half of the night Rebound increase of REM sleep in the second half of the night with increased arousals

Insomnia

Possible Causes of Insomnia

Primary sleep disorders	Primary insomnia
	Narcolepsy
	Obstructive sleep apnea
	Circadian rhythm, sleep disorder
	Periodic limb movement disorder
	Brief, stereotypic, nonepileptiform movement of the limbs, which increases with age
	Can occur in association with folate deficiency, renal disease, anemia, and the use of antidepressants
	Nocturnal myoclonus
	Repetitive, brief leg jerks that are associated with transient awakenings leading to sleep fragmentation
	Associated with sleep apnea, narcolepsy, uremia, diabetes, and central nervous system disorders
	Restless leg syndrome
	Characterized by the irresistible urge to move the legs/crawling feelings at rest or while trying to fall asleep
	Associated with anemia, pregnancy, nocturnal myoclonus and with uremia
	Parasomnias (e.g., night terrors, sleepwalking)
Psychiatric	Anxiety disorders
	Affective disorders
	Psychosis
	Substance or alcohol abuse
	Eating disorders
	Dementia
	Psychological stress
	Bedtime worrying
	Poor sleep hygiene/conditioning (associating the bed with wakefulness)
Medical	Pain from any source or cause (e.g., arthritis, back pain)
	Dyspnea from any cause (e.g., asthma, chronic obstructive pulmonary disease, congestive heart failure)
	Gastrointestinal disease (e.g., gastroesophageal reflux disease)
	Neurologic disease (Parkinson, Alzheimer)
	Nocturia (e.g., uncontrolled diabetes, benign prostatic hypertrophy)
	Menopause
	Drug or alcohol intoxication or withdrawal
Medication-induced	Serotonin reuptake inhibitors
	Monoamine oxidase inhibitors
	Buproprion
	Stimulants (e.g., Ritalin)
	Short-acting hypnotics
	Beta-blockers
	Bronchodilators
	Corticosteroids
	Theophylline
	Thyroid hormones
	Caffeine
	Nicotine

Evaluation

- Perform a thorough medical and psychiatric history (including history of substance abuse).
- Question patient about his or her routine sleep-wake habits.
- Have patient perform a 2-week sleep-wake log to include the following information:
  - Irregular sleep-wake patterns, including number of arousals.
  - Perceived length of sleep time and its relationship to daytime mood and alertness.
  - Napping.
  - Use of stimulants, hypnotics, or alcohol.
  - Diet, including the timing of meals.
  - Activity and exercise during the day.
- Inquire about symptoms suggestive of a primary sleep disorder (e.g. sleep apnea) and/or medical etiologies (e.g. nocturnal incontinence or polyuria, orthopnea, paroxysmal nocturnal dyspnea).
- Question carefully about falling asleep while driving or while performing any other potentially dangerous activity.
- Obtain collateral information from partners, such as snoring, respiratory pauses longer than 10 seconds, jerking, unusual body movements, or somnambulism.
- Consider referral to a sleep disorder clinic.

Management of Insomnia
Behavioral Treatments

Sleep hygiene	Maintain a regular sleep-wake routine, including waking at the same time 7 days a week.
	Ensure a comfortable sleep environment that is noise free, dark, and well ventilated.
	Use the bedroom only for sleeping and for sexual activity. If unable to sleep, get out of bed and engage in another activity.
	Return to bed when sleepy.
	Get a steady daily amount of exercise, but avoid vigorous exercise 4 h before bed.
	A light snack before bedtime may be helpful.
	Do not eat a heavy meal close to bedtime and reduce liquid intake in the evening if possible.
	Avoid caffeine 4 h before bedtime.
	Quit smoking or avoid smoking near bedtime.
	Avoid ongoing use of alcohol and recreational drugs.
	Avoid daytime naps.
Relaxation training	Progressive relaxation, breathing exercises (or yoga), biofeedback, and guided visualization.
Stimulus control therapy	Attempt to foster stimulus cues for sleeping and decrease bedroom stimulus associations with sleeplessness.

(Continued)

	Goal is to associate the bed and bedroom with rapid sleep onset.
Sleep restriction therapy	Sleep schedule is compressed to the actual time spent sleeping then gradually increased as sleep efficiency increases.
	Advise patients to exercise extreme care, especially when performing potentially dangerous actions (e.g., driving) during this therapy.
Bright light therapy	Seeks to reset the biological clock through precise timing of bright light exposure.

Pharmacologic Management

Medication	Onset	Dose (mg)	Special Considerations
Benzodiazepines			Use of benzodiazepines has been associated with daytime sedation, impaired cognitive and psychomotor function, memory impairment, and risk of tolerance and dependence.
Flurazepam (Dalmane)	Rapid	15, 30	Long half-life may lead to daytime sedation.
Temazepam (Restoril)	Intermediate	7.5, 15	Short duration of action limits daytime sedation. Rebound insomnia. Preferred agent in presence of hepatic dysfunction.
Triazolam (Halcion)	Rapid	0.125, 0.25, 0.50	Useful with sleep initiation. Rebound insomnia and anxiety. Reports of dose-related anterograde amnesia.
Newer hypnotics			
Zolpidem (Ambien)	Rapid	5, 10	Case reports of sleepwalking, hallucinatory phenomenon and other sensory distortions, anterograde amnesia. Useful for initiation of sleep.
Zaleplon (Sonata)	Rapid	5, 10, 20	Useful for initiation of sleep. Anterograde amnesia.
Eszopiclone (Lunesta)	30–60 min	1, 2, 3	Useful for initiation of sleep. High doses may cause amnesia, elevated mood, and psychotic symptoms.
Ramelteon (Rozerem)	30–60 min	8	Newer drug with limited evidence-based clinical data available.

(*Continued*)

Medication	Onset	Dose (mg)	Special Considerations
			Adverse effects reported include dizziness, headache, worsening insomnia, sedation, fatigue.
Antidepressants			
Amitriptyline	10–50 h	10, 25, 50, 75, 100, 125, 150	Drowsiness, confusion, anticholinergic effects, increased risk of falls, orthostatic hypotension, cardiac conduction defects. Lower dose typically used for treatment of insomnia.
Trazodone	4–9 h	50, 100, 150, 300	Drowsiness, priapism, orthostatic hypotension, cardiac conduction defects, weight gain, seizure risk, headaches.
Antipsychotics			
Quetiapine	6 h	25, 50, 100, 150, 200, 300	Extrapyramidal effects, sedation, orthostatic hypotension, weight gain, increased risk of falls.
Miscellaneous			
Diphenhydramine	1–4 h	25, 50	Anticholinergic effects, sedation, incoordination, increased risk of falls, cognitive impairment, risk of delirium in elderly.

Source: Adapted from Hales RE, Yudofsky SC. *The American Psychiatric Publishing Textbook of Clinical Psychiatry.* 4th ed. Washington, DC: American Psychiatric Publishing, Inc; 2003:978–979.

References

Benca RM. Diagnosis and treatment of chronic insomnia: A review. *Psychiatric Services.* March 2005:332–340.

Hales RE, Yudofsky SC. *The American Psychiatric Publishing Textbook of Clinical Psychiatry.* 4th ed. Washington, DC: American Psychiatric Publishing Inc; 2003:975–991.

Shatzberg AF, Nemeroff CB, eds. *The American Psychiatric Publishing Textbook of Psychopharmacology.* 3rd ed. Arlington, VA: American Psychiatric Publishing Inc; 2004:1154.

Yudofsky SC, Hales RE. *Essentials of Neuropsychiatry and Clinical Neurosciences.* Washington, DC: American Psychiatric Publishing Inc; 2004:315–336.

Chapter 35

TRAUMATIC BRAIN INJURY

Epidemiology

- Most common cause of death among persons under age 35 are injuries incurred during motor vehicle accidents.
- In the United States, between 2.5 million and 6.5 million individuals live with the long-term consequences of traumatic brain injury (TBI).

Neuropsychiatric Assessment of Traumatic Brain Injury

History Taking

- Involvement in situations associated with head trauma, such as motor vehicle accidents, assaults, sports.
- Any alteration in consciousness, including feeling dazed or confused, loss of consciousness, or amnesic periods.
- Hospitalization and/or presence of posttraumatic symptoms, such as headache, dizziness, irritability, problems with concentration, and sensitivity to noise or light.
- Differentiate between loss of consciousness and posttraumatic amnesia, as patient may attribute difficulty in recalling events to being unconscious.
- Collateral information from family members about the effects of the injury on the behavior of the patient.

Evaluation

- Computed tomography (CT) is useful for detecting contusions, hematomas, and fractures. However, initial CT evaluations may not detect lesions in the acute phase.
- Magnetic resonance imaging (MRI) is more sensitive in detecting lesions in the acute phase, particularly lesions in the frontal and temporal lobes.
- Electroencephalography as indicated to detect the presence of seizures or abnormal areas of functioning.
- Consider neuropsychological testing to document cognitive and intellectual deficits.

Neuropsychiatric Manifestation	Clinical Feature

Personality changes	Problematic behavioral traits prominent before TBI become more pronounced, with a 2- to 3-fold increased prevalence of personality disorders after TBI.
	The most common disorders are borderline, avoidant, paranoid, obsessive compulsive, and narcissistic.
	Frontal lobe syndrome:
	  Impaired social judgment, labile affect, uncharacteristic lewdness, decreased grooming and hygiene, with intact cognition.
	Orbitofrontal syndrome:
	  Behavioral excesses such as impulsivity, disinhibition, hyperactivity, distractibility, and mood lability.
	Dorsolateral frontal cortex:
	  Slowness, apathy, and perseveration.
	Inferior orbital surface of the frontal and anterior temporal lobes:
	  Outbursts of rage and violent behavior.

Intellectual changes	Impairments in attention, language, memory, concentration, and executive function. Increased risk of Alzheimer disease and shorter time to onset of Alzheimer disease for those at risk. Behavioral and learning problems in children.
Psychiatric disorders	Increased incidence of major depression, dysthymia, anxiety disorders, including posttraumatic stress disorder and generalized anxiety disorder, and drug abuse and dependence.
Suicide	Increased risk of suicidality and suicide attempts, possibly due to the combination of major depression with disinhibition secondary to frontal lobe injury.
Delirium	Although delirium is most often due to injury to brain tissue, it is important to evaluate for other causes such as medications, substance withdrawal, or other medical causes (refer to Chapter 30).
Posttraumatic epilepsy	Increased risk of repeated seizures subsequent to TBI. Risk increases with severe head injury, penetrating head trauma, premorbid alcohol use, and intracranial hemorrhage.
Sleep disorders	Disrupted sleep patterns, including hypersomnia and sleep-disordered breathing.
Postconcussion syndrome	Syndrome recognized by the DSM-IV-TR[a] as consisting of research criteria encompassing somatic (headache, dizziness, fatigue, insomnia), cognitive, perceptual (tinnitus, sensitivity to noise and light), and emotional symptoms.
Aggression	Increased risk of agitation and violent behaviors that are typically reactive, impulsive, and nonpurposeful.

[a]*Diagnostic and Statistical Manual of Mental Disorders*. 4th ed. Text revision. Washington, DC: American Psychiatric Association; 2000.

Management of Traumatic Brain Injury
General Considerations

- Raise and lower doses of psychiatric medications in small increments gradually due to sensitivity to side effects of psychotropics.
- Initiate psychotropic drug at lowest dosages and titrate as needed to address symptoms while minimizing adverse effects.
- Ensure an adequate trial of psychotropic drug with respect to dosage and duration of treatment.
- Frequently monitor the patient's clinical status to assess continued need for medications prescribed and to minimize the risk of polypharmacy.

Target Symptoms	Suggested Medications	Considerations in Selecting Drug
Depression Emotional "incontinence"	Fluoxetine Sertraline Citalopram	Choose drugs with the fewest sedative, hypotensive, and anticholinergic side effects. Avoid drugs that lower seizure threshold, such as bupropion.
Mania	Valproic acid Lamotrigine	Caution with lithium carbonate due to risk of confusion and lowering seizure threshold. Patients with brain injury are at increased risk for these adverse effects.
Attention Fatigue	Dextroamphetamine Methylphenidate	Can improve the rate of recovery, but not the extent of recovery. May lead to paranoia, dysphoria, agitation, and irritability.
Apathy	Bromocriptine Amantadine	Bromocriptine can cause sedation, psychosis, headaches, and delirium. Amantadine may cause confusion, hallucinations, edema, and hypotension.
Cognition	Donepezil	May cause sedation, insomnia, dizziness, diarrhea, and bradycardia.
Psychosis	Risperidone	Can cause hypotension, sedation, confusion, and extrapyramidal symptoms.
Acute aggression and agitation	Olanzapine Quetiapine	Extreme caution with clozapine due to significant dose-related incidence of seizures.

(Continued)

Target Symptoms	Suggested Medications	Considerations in Selecting Drug
Chronic aggression	Atypical antipsychotics Valproic acid Beta-blockers (propranolol)	Monitor for bradycardia and hypotension when using beta-blockers. Do not use concurrently with thioridazine.
Sleep	Trazodone	Nonpharmacologic approaches preferred before considering medications. Side effect of hypotension.
Seizures	Valproic acid Carbamazepine	Drugs of choice for patients with aggressive episodes with comorbid seizure disorder. Ensure primary management of seizure disorder by neurologist.

References

Daniel JP. Traumatic brain injury: Choosing drugs to assist recovery. *Curr Psychiatr.* 5(5):57–68.

Yudofsky SC, Hales RE. *Essentials of Neuropsychiatry and Clinical Neurosciences.* Arlington, VA: American Psychiatric Publishing, Inc; 2004:241–291.

Chapter 36
HIV/AIDS

Pretest HIV Counseling[1]

1. Discussion of HIV test, including risks and benefits, sensitivity and specificity, possible need for confirmatory testing.
2. Discuss meaning of a positive result and clarify distortions (e.g., the test detects exposure to the AIDS virus; it is not a test for AIDS).
3. Discuss the meaning of a negative result (e.g., seroconversion requires time, recent high-risk behavior may require follow-up testing).
4. Plans for dealing with a positive or negative test result.
5. Be available to discuss the patient's fears and concerns.
6. Discuss why the test is necessary.
7. Explore the patient's potential reactions to a positive result. Take appropriate necessary steps to intervene in a potentially catastrophic reaction. Carefully assess support systems.
8. Discuss the confidentiality issues relevant to the testing situation, including limits to confidentiality such as potential for others to be harmed.
   - Discuss who has access to the test results, including state mandatory reporting regulations. Be aware that reporting guidelines vary from state to state.
   - All states have mandatory name reporting when a patient is diagnosed with AIDS.
   - Some states mandate reporting the names of individuals who test HIV positive.
9. Discuss with the patient how being seropositive can potentially affect social status (e.g., health and life insurance coverage, employment, housing).
10. Explore high-risk behaviors and recommend risk-reducing interventions.
11. Where to obtain further information or, if applicable, HIV prevention counseling.
12. Document discussions in chart.
13. Allow the patient time to ask questions.

Posttest HIV Counseling

1. Interpretation of test result:
   - Clarify distortion (e.g., "a negative test still means you could contract the virus at a future time; it does not mean you are immune from AIDS").

---

[1]. Information on pre- and posttest HIV counseling in this and the next section is modified, with permission, from Rosse RB, Giese AA, Deutsch SI, Morihisa JM. *Laboratory and Diagnostic Testing in Psychiatry*. Washington, DC: American Psychiatric Press; 1989:55,58.

- Ask questions about the patient's understanding and emotional reaction to the test result.
2. Recommendations for prevention of transmission (careful discussion of high-risk behaviors and guidelines for prevention of transmission).
3. Recommendations on the follow-up of sexual partners and needle contacts.
   - Strongly encourage patient to inform current, previous, and prospective sex partners or persons with whom needles were shared of their infection with HIV, so appropriate precautions can be taken. If a patient has not disclosed their HIV-positive status to a partner and continues high-risk behavior, it may be ethical to notify identifiable sexual partners or other at-risk individuals. However, it may not be legally permissible and psychiatrists should consult with risk management before breaching confidentiality.
4. Women who are pregnant or desiring pregnancy should seek counseling and specialized medical care from a specialist.
5. Inform physicians, dentists, and other health care providers of their HIV status to ensure specialized medical care and that appropriate precautions are taken.
6. If test result is positive, recommendations against donating blood, sperm, or organs and against sharing razors, toothbrushes, and anything else that may have blood on it.
7. Referral for appropriate psychological support:
   - HIV-positive patients often need access to a mental health team (assess need for inpatient versus outpatient care; consider individual or group supportive therapy). Common themes include the shock of the diagnosis, the fear of death, and social consequences, grief over potential losses, and dashed hopes for good news.
   - Also look for depression, hopelessness, anger, frustration, guilt, and obsessional themes.
   - Activate supports available to the patient (e.g., family, friends, and community services).

Neuropsychiatric Assessment of a Patient with HIV/AIDS

History Taking

- Psychiatric history, with special emphasis on suicidality and current emotional state.
- Sexual and substance abuse history.
- Past medical history, including new onset of medical and neurologic symptoms.
- Social history, including social support and religious beliefs.
- Knowledge about HIV and AIDS.

HIV/AIDS Psychiatric Syndromes and Management

General Considerations

- Protease inhibitors are metabolized by the hepatic cytochrome P450 oxidase system (especially 3A4 and 2D6) and can therefore increase

levels of certain psychotropic drugs that are similarly metabolized, including bupropion, meperidine, methadone, various benzodiazepines, antipsychotics, and antidepressants.
- When indicated, prescribe all psychotropics cautiously, including using lower dosages and titrating slowly.
- Consider medication risks to avoid adverse effects, such as leucopenia from carbamazepine.
- Be aware of drug metabolism/clearance pathways and end-organ effects to minimize drug–drug interactions.
- Promote adherence to all medications as even minor deviations from prescribed regimens can result in loss of efficacy and developing viral resistance.
- Psychotherapy (e.g., cognitive behavioral, psychodynamic, interpersonal, psychoeducational) has been found to be more effective in combination with psychopharmacology than psychopharmacology alone.
- Coordinate care with patient's HIV/AIDS provider.

Neuropsychiatric Manifestation	Clinical Feature	Management
HIV-associated dementia	Subcortical type of dementia Progressive cognitive decline (such as impaired verbal memory and learning, impaired executive functioning), motor dysfunction, and behavioral abnormalities Significant functional impairment Poor prognostic sign	When indicated, use atypical antipsychotics with a low risk of extrapyramidal side effects due to increased sensitivity to extrapyramidal side effects
Mild neurocognitive disorder	Neurocognitive impairment in two domains Mild functional impairment	Complete medical/neurological evaluation Formal neuropsychological testing can help fully document dysfunction and identify areas of strength
Delirium/altered mental status	Most common causes are iatrogenic, infection, neoplasms, and metabolic disturbances	Repeat complete medical/neurological evaluation O_2 saturation/arterial blood gas analysis if indicated Labs: complete blood cell count with differential, CHEM 7, Venereal Disease Research

(Continued)

Neuropsychiatric Manifestation	Clinical Feature	Management
		Laboratory test (VDRL), vitamin B_{12}, folate, CD4 count and viral load test, toxicology screen
		Brain imaging to rule out space-occupying lesion
		Lumbar puncture if indicated
Anxiety	Commonly generalized anxiety disorder, posttraumatic stress disorder, and obsessive compulsive disorder	Avoid benzodiazepines due to drug–drug interactions
Depression	Associated with accelerated HIV disease progression and noncompliance with treatment	Mirtazapine, citalopram, and sustained-release bupropion are effective and have low risk of drug–drug interactions
		Selective serotonin reuptake inhibitors generally well tolerated, but risk of serotonin syndrome due to cytochrome P450 2D6 inhibition
		Due to likely interaction with antiretroviral regimen, caution with selection and dosing of antidepressant
Mania	Most commonly in late-stage disease complicated by neurocognitive impairment	Divalproex sodium has been found to be helpful and well tolerated in HIV patients on antiretroviral therapy
		Monitor hepatic function closely
Substance abuse	Prevalent among individuals with or at risk for HIV infection	Treatment a priority as active substance use is associated with high-risk behaviors
	Comorbid psychiatric disorders include anxiety, depression, and psychosis	Care should encompass multidisciplinary, structured intervention
Suicide	Factors that may increase suicidality include recent death of friends due to AIDS, recent positive HIV test, clinical deterioration, social issues, inadequate	Perform suicide assessment as indicated
		Monitor closely during periods of increased risk for suicidality
		Refer for appropriate psychological support, such as peer support

(Continued)

Neuropsychiatric Manifestation	Clinical Feature	Management
	social and financial support, and dementia or delirium	groups, individual counseling Activate supports available to the patient Hospitalize if necessary
Psychosis	Late-stage complication	Repeat complete medical/neurological evaluation and workup, particularly for new-onset psychosis Atypical antipsychotics are generally well tolerated, but caution due to risk of metabolic syndrome and increased susceptibility to extrapyramidal symptoms Avoid depot antipsychotics in advanced HIV disease

Neuropsychiatric Side Effects of Selected Medications Used in HIV Disease

Drug	Target Illness	Side Effects
Acyclovir	Herpes encephalitis	Visual hallucinations, depersonalization, tearfulness, confusion, hyperesthesia, hyperacusis, thought insertion, insomnia
Amphotericin B	Cryptococcosis	Delirium, peripheral neuropathy, diplopia
Atazanavir	HIV	Depression, headache
β-Lactam antibiotics	Infections	Confusion, paranoia, hallucinations, mania, coma
Co-trimoxazole	*Pneumocystis carinii* pneumonia	Depression, loss of appetite, insomnia, apathy
Cycloserine	Tuberculosis	Psychosis, somnolence, depression, confusion, tremor, vertigo, paresis, seizures, dysarthria
Delavirdine	HIV	Anxiety, depression, insomnia, headache
Didanosine	HIV	Nervousness, anxiety, confusions, seizures, insomnia, peripheral neuropathy
Efavirenz	HIV	Nightmares, depression, confusion, ataxia, and vertigo-like symptoms

(Continued)

Drug	Target Illness	Side Effects
Fosamprenavir	HIV	Headache, oral paresthesia, depression or other mood disorders
Foscarnet	Cytomegalovirus	Paresthesias, seizures, headache, irritability, hallucinations, confusion
Interferon-α	Kaposi's sarcoma	Depression, weakness, headache, myalgias, confusion
Isoniazid	Tuberculosis	Depression, agitation, hallucinations, paranoia, impaired memory, anxiety
Lamivudine	HIV	Insomnia, mania
Methotrexate	Lymphoma	Encephalopathy (at high dose)
Pentamidine	*Pneumocystis carinii* pneumonia	Confusion, anxiety, lability, hallucinations
Procarbazine	Lymphoma	Mania, loss of appetite, insomnia, nightmares, confusion, malaise
Quinolones	Infection	Psychosis, delirium, seizures, anxiety, insomnia, depression
Stavudine	HIV	Headache, asthenia, malaise, confusion, depression, seizures, excitability, anxiety, mania, early morning awakening, insomnia
Sulfonamides	Infection	Psychosis, delirium, confusion, depression, hallucinations
Thiabendazole	Strongyloidiasis	Hallucinations, olfactory disturbance
Vinblastine	Kaposi's sarcoma	Depression, loss of appetite, headache
Vincristine	Kaposi's sarcoma	Hallucinations, headache, ataxia, sensory loss
Zalcitabine	HIV	Headache, confusion, impaired concentration, somnolence, asthenia, depression, seizures, peripheral neuropathy
Zidovudine	HIV	Headache, malaise, asthenia, insomnia, unusually vivid dreams, restlessness, severe agitation, mania, auditory hallucinations, confusion

Reprinted, with permission, from American Psychiatric Association Steering Committee on Practice Guidelines. Appendix C. Neuropsychiatric side effects of selected medications used in HIV disease. In *Quick Reference to the American Psychiatric Association Practice Guidelines for the Treatment of Psychiatric Disorders, Compendium 2006.* Arlington, VA: American Psychiatric Association; 2006:70–71.

References

American Psychiatric Association Steering Committee on Practice Guidelines. *American Psychiatric Association Practice Guidelines for the Treatment of Psychiatric Disorders, Compendium 2006.* Arlington, VA: American Psychiatric Association; 2006:169–261.

Horwarth E, Nash S. Psychiatric manifestations of HIV infection and AIDS. *Psychiatric Times.* November 2005:34–36.

Quick Reference to the American Psychiatric Association Practice Guidelines for the Treatment of Psychiatric Disorders, Compendium 2006. Arlington, VA: American Psychiatric Association; 2006:49–74.

Yudofsky SC, Hales RE. *Essentials of Neuropsychiatry and Clinical Neurosciences.* Arlington, VA: American Psychiatric Publishing, Inc; 2004:371–379.

Section IV

Psychiatry

Chapter 37

VIOLENCE

Assessing Risk Factors for Violence

Dynamic	Static
Homicidal plan	Past crime/violence
Weapon access	Impulsivity
Drug intoxication	Antisocial/borderline
Command auditory hallucinations	Childhood abuse (e.g., violence at home)
Paranoid delusions	Disinhibition secondary to delirium/dementia

Premeditated/chronic
  Presence of a victim
  Frequent and open threats
  Concrete plan
	Male ages 15–24

Visible agitation	Early loss of parent
Mania	Current suicidal behavior/history of suicide attempts

General Considerations for Evaluation and Management of an Agitated Patient

- Quick search of patient for potential weapons upon arrival in unit.
- Consider and attempt to rule out any medical etiology for agitation necessitating urgent management (e.g., delirium tremens).
- Maintain the safety of the patient, staff, and other patients at all times.
- Monitor closely for signs of pre-escalation, such as:
  - Pacing
  - Verbal threats
- Appearance of escalating psychotic symptoms
- In the presence of escalating agitation, assemble adequate trained personnel prior to speaking with patient.
- Attempt to de-escalate patient by offering oral medication and/or offering a voluntary time out in a quiet, secluded area.
- While speaking with the patient, avoid direct eye contact and address patient in a nonprovocative manner.
- Maintain a nonthreatening posture and safe distance from the patient.
- Before approaching patient, check for any items that can potentially be used as weapons (e.g., pens, ties).
- Clearly explain procedure to patient, that he or she will not be harmed, and its necessity for maintaining everyone's safety.

- Allow the patient to walk to the seclusion area voluntarily before escorting forcefully.
- Monitor patient closely and be prepared to administer emergent IM medication and perform restraint in the event of violent behavior.
- Remove restraints sequentially.
- Clearly delineate behaviors that must be observed prior to discontinuation of seclusion and/or restraint (e.g., patient sitting quietly in an unlocked seclusion room).

Indications for Seclusion and Restraint
- Danger to others/self.
- Credible verbal and physical threats.
- Disruption of the treatment milieu.
- Not responding to verbal intervention or redirection.

Risk Management Guidelines for Seclusion and Restraint
- Review and follow written guidelines of the institution.
- Physician should see the patient within 1 h of seclusion/restraint to evaluate for efficacy of emergent medication(s), improvement in behaviors necessitating seclusion/restraint, and cursory mental status/physical exam to include vital signs.
- Continue above monitoring every 4 h and renew order if necessary (2 h for children/adolescents).
- Review state/institution rules and regulations that may differ from above guidelines.

Documentation Guidelines for Seclusion and Restraint
- Date/time of evaluation.
- Reasons for seclusion/restraint.
- Steps taken to attempt to prevent seclusion/restraint.
- Evaluation of patient, including mental status exam.
- Examination of patient, including mental status exam.
- Documentation of any injuries incurred.
- Criteria for graded discontinuation of seclusion/restraint.

Emergency Medication

Caution must be used in administering neuroleptics because they can lower the seizure threshold.

Agent	Dosage	Special Considerations
Lorazepam	1–2 mg IM or orally. Repeat q hour if IM or q 4–6 h if oral.	Maximum daily dose of 10 mg/d. No active metabolites. Watch for paradoxical agitation in older, delirious patients and children. Watch for respiratory depression.
Haloperidol	2–10 mg IM q4h with maximum daily dose of 20 mg.	Use with Benadryl to prevent acute dystonia. Caution in delirium and alcohol/drug toxicity or withdrawal (can lower seizure threshold).
Olanzapine	5–10 mg IM. Repeat dose of 10 mg can be given in 4 h. Lower in elderly (2.5–5 mg).	Available in oral dissolvable tab.
Chlorpromazine	25 mg IM q4h with increased dose over 1–3 d.	Caution in delirium and alcohol/drug toxicity or withdrawal. Caution due to risk of postural hypotension and QTc prolongation.
Ziprasidone	Oral: 40 mg p.o. BID (with food), increase to 80 mg p.o. BID. IM: 10–20 mg initially, then 10 mg q2h.	Maximum of 40 mg IM/d. Do not use with recent myocardial infarction or uncompensated congestive heart failure (Ejection Fraction <30%). Caution with QTc prolongation.
Valproate	20–30 mg/kg/d.	Also available in liquid/IV form. With Depakote ER need 8%–20% higher dose, e.g., add 250 mg/d to current dose. Target serum level → 50–125 µg/ml.

Long-Term Medication

Pharmacotherapy, including the use of selective serotonin reuptake inhibitors, scheduled antipsychotics, mood stabilizers, long half-life benzodiazepines, and propranolol (e.g., 20 mg BID-TID with holding parameters and caution with bronchial asthma, chronic obstructive pulmonary disease) has demonstrated efficacy with treatment of aggressive behavior in affectively under-controlled individuals.

Duty to Protect: *Tarasoff v. University of California Regents*

Tarasoff 1—Duty to warn.
Tarasoff 2—Duty to protect.

Of note, interpretation of *Tarasoff* ruling varies from state to state. Applies when there is a serious threat of harm to an identifiable person(s). May also include threats communicated by the patient to a credible third party, such as a family member or close acquaintance of the patient, and when the psychotherapist or a treatment team staff person is subsequently notified or informed of the serious threat made by the patient.

1. Warn the individual you believe to be in danger, by telephone and in writing (send certified mail, return receipt).
2. Notify the police who cover the jurisdiction of the person in danger, by telephone and in writing.
3. Take steps to have the patient hospitalized on a 5150 for danger to others.
4. Tell the patient who presents the danger about warning the potential victim.
5. Be aware that unlike child abuse reporting, there is no immunity for clinicians from legal liability for violating confidentiality in warnings without merit.

References

Garcia KS, Lin TL. *Washington Manual Psychiatry Survival Guide.* St Louis: Lippincott Williams & Wilkins; 2003:144.

Hales RE, Yudofsky SC, eds. *The American Psychiatric Publishing Textbook of Clinical Psychiatry.* Washington, DC: American Psychiatric Publishing, Inc; 2003:1485–1505.

Tasman A, Kay J, Lieberman JA. *Psychiatry Therapeutics.* 2nd ed. New York: John Wiley & Sons; 2003:442.

Chapter 38

CAPACITY

Capacity Assessment	

When to assess capacity	Abrupt change in mental status
	Refusal of recommended treatment
	  Not willing to discuss refusal
	  Reasons for refusal not clear
	  Refusal based on misinformation or irrational biases
	Hastily consenting to risky or invasive treatment without careful consideration of risks or benefits
	Known risk factor for impaired decision making
	  Chronic neurologic or psychiatric condition
	  Significant cultural or language barrier
	  Educational level
	  Acknowledged fear or discomfort with institutional health care settings
	  Adolescents younger than 18 years or adults older than 85 years

How to assess capacity	Components
	  When consulted:
	    Confirm that informed consent was attempted and patient given adequate information
	    Request for capacity is task specific
	  Directed clinical interview (see below)
	  Collateral from other clinicians and caregivers
	  Screening for depression and/or suicidality
	  Screening for psychosis
	  Screening for altered mental status/delirium
	    Physical assessment
	    Laboratory evaluation and studies, particularly to rule out reversible causes of altered mental status
	  Screening for cognitive impairment
	    Mini-mental state exam (MMSE)
	Directed clinical interview
	1. Determine ability of patient to understand treatment and proposed care options and how they apply this information to their own situation
	  Understanding of their condition
	  What specific test or treatment has their doctor recommended
	  Whether they think the specific test or treatment is best for them and reasons for and against
	  Understanding of the benefits of treatment and what are the odds that the treatment will work for them
	  Understanding of the risks of treatment and what are the odds that they may have a side effect or bad outcome
	  Understanding of outcome if nothing done
	  Understanding of outcome if treatment accepted
	  Understanding of any alternatives to proposed treatment

Capacity Assessment	
	2. Determine ability of patient to reason with above information in a manner that is supported by the facts and the patient's own values
	What factors/issues are important to patient in deciding about their treatment
	Does patient trust doctor? Why or why not?
	3. Determine ability of patient to communicate and express a choice clearly
Formal assessment tools	Aid to Capacity Evaluation (ACE)
	MacArthur Competence Assessment Tool (MacCAT)
Who should assess capacity?	Primary care physicians are qualified to perform capacity assessments
	Psychiatry consultation
Patients lacking capacity	When appropriate, intervention to restore reversible causes of lack of capacity, such as altered mental status/delirium, acute psychiatric illness
	A determination of whether surrogacy will be necessary
	Bioethics panel and/or risk management for complicated cases

References

Hillard R, Zitek B. *Emergency Psychiatry.* McGraw-Hill Company; 2004:51–53.

Tunzi M. Can the patient decide? Evaluating patient capacity in practice. *American Family Physician.* 2001;64(2)299–306.

Chapter 39

ALCOHOL INTOXICATION AND WITHDRAWAL

Intoxication

Blood Alcohol Level (BAL)

Alcohol is metabolized at a rate of ~30 mg/dl/h, dependent on tolerance and liver function.

BAL(mg/dl)	Clinical Features
30	Attention difficulties (mild), euphoria
50	Coordination problems
100	Ataxia, drunk driving
200	Confusion, decreased consciousness
>400	Anesthesia, coma, death

Withdrawal

Time of Onset	Syndrome	Clinical Features
6–8 h	Minor withdrawal	Tremulousness/"shakes," mild anxiety, headache, diaphoresis, palpitations, anorexia, gastrointestinal upset.
8–12 h	Alcoholic hallucinosis	Psychotic or perceptual symptoms.
12–24 h	Seizures	10% of all chronic drinkers endure a grand mal seizure, with 1/3 progressing to delirium tremens. Status epilepticus uncommon; however, there may be more than one seizure 3–6 h after the first seizure.
72 h–1 week	Delirium tremens	Autonomic instability, mild fever, insomnia. Hallucinations may be auditory of a persecutory nature or tactile. Fatality <1%. Cause of death usually infectious fat emboli or cardiac arrhythmias.

Note: Not uncommon for patient to skip a stage and proceed from tremulousness to delirium tremens.

Criteria for Hospitalization/Intensive Care Unit Observation of the Withdrawing Alcoholic[1]

1. Severe tremulousness, other autonomic symptoms, or hallucinosis.
2. Significant volume depletion, acid-base or electrolyte disturbance.
3. Fever and delirium or seizure.
4. Fever above 38.1°C (100.5°F).
5. First seizure ever or seizure without prior evaluation.
6. Delirium.
7. History of alcohol withdrawal delirium.
8. Wernicke encephalopathy (e.g., ataxia, nystagmus, internuclear ophthalmoplegia).
9. Head trauma with loss of consciousness.
10. Failure to respond to initial outpatient treatment.
11. Presence of significant comorbidity requiring hospitalization.
    - Decompensated liver disease
    - Respiratory compromise or failure
    - Pneumonia
    - Gastrointestinal bleeding
    - Pancreatitis
    - Severe malnutrition
    - Angina
    - Multiple seizures, particularly with incomplete recovery
    - Unstable psychiatric illness, such as severe depression, suicide risk, active schizophrenia, or bipolar disorder
12. Need for pharmacologic management with inability to take appropriately as an outpatient.
    - No responsible other person available to help with medication
    - No health care services available to manage as outpatient
13. Although not absolutely required, strongly consider hospitalization for the elderly and for those withdrawing with a blood alcohol level of 150 mg/dl or greater.

Sample Inpatient Orders

1. Monitor vital signs q4h while in withdrawal, then q8h × 24 h, then qd. Also monitor vital signs prn as indicated by severity of withdrawal.
2. Call physician for temperature >100°F, heart rate >110, blood pressure >160/90 or <90/60, respiratory rate >24 or <12, hallucinations not responding to treatment, and/or change in mental status.
3. Call physician for seizures.
4. Call physician for delirium or altered sensorium.
5. Routine meds
   - Thiamine 100 mg IM × 3d then 100 mg p.o. qd.

---

1. Reprinted from Shader RI. *Manual of Psychiatric Therapeutics*. 3rd ed. Philadelphia: Lippincott Williams & Wilkins; 2003:149 (Table 12.4). With permission.

- MVI with minerals p.o. qd.
- $MgSO_4$ 500 mg p.o. qd.
- Zinc gluconate 50 mg p.o. qd for 5 d.
- Pepcid 20 mg p.o. BID.

6. Mild withdrawal (systolic blood pressure >150, diastolic blood pressure >90, heart rate >100, temperature >100°F on presentation)
   - Librium 25/50 mg q4h prn shakes or insomnia.
   - OR Valium 5/10 mg q4h prn.
   - OR lorazepam 2 mg q4h prn.
7. Moderate withdrawal (with agitation, tremulousness, or insomnia and blood pressure >150/95 or heart rate >100 or temperature >100°F)
   - Librium 50 mg p.o. q6h and Librium___mg p.o. q2h prn (maximum 400 mg/24 h). (If excess sedation or blood pressure <90/60, decrease Librium dose to 25 mg.)
   - OR Valium 10 mg p.o. or IM q6h and ___mg p.o. q2h prn (maximum 100 mg/24 h). (Lower dose to 5 mg if excess sedation or blood pressure <90/60.)
   - OR for liver disease or age 65+, lorazepam 1mg q6h and ___mg p.o. q2h prn. (Lower dose to 0.5 mg if excess sedation or blood pressure <90/60.)
8. Count total dose needed for stabilization of signs.
9. Total divided by 4 is amount to give four times a day.
10. When indicated, taper daily total about 25% over 3 d, continue no more than 10 d.
11. Adjunct meds
    - Haldol 0.5–2 mg p.o. or IM q2h prn agitation/perceptual disturbances. Be cautious in using antipsychotic medications as they reduce the seizure threshold. Avoid conventional antipsychotics, such as chlorpromazine and thioridazine that cause hypotension.
    - Atenolol 50 mg p.o. qd prn heart rate >100, autonomic hyperactivity OR propranolol 10 mg p.o. q6h prn autonomic symptoms. (Propranolol contraindicated in patients with asthma, insulin-dependent diabetes, congestive heart failure.) OR clonidine 0.1–0.3 mg BID-TID prn. For above, hold if systolic blood pressure <90, diastolic blood pressure <60, or heart rate <60. Above meds do not protect from seizures and delirium.
12. Medical workup for alcohol withdrawal
    - Laboratory: blood alcohol level (if alert and oriented at high alcohol levels, patient is very tolerant and more likely to withdraw), complete blood cell count with differential, CHEM 7, Ca, Mg, PO_4, hepatic function, GGT, albumin, total protein, PT, lipid panel, Hep BsAg, B_{12}, folate, stool guaic, urinalysis, serum and urine toxicology screens, serum amylase, HIV test.
    - Imaging: chest x-ray, EKG, head CT if indicated.
13. If possible, avoid physical restraints.

Outpatient Management[2]

1. History, physical, and laboratory evaluation to look for indications for hospitalization and co-occurring disorders.
2. Intramuscular thiamine, 100 mg, followed by daily multivitamin, folate 1 mg p.o. qd, thiamine 100 mg p.o. qd.
3. Initial dose of benzodiazepine (chlordiazepoxide 50–100 mg p.o.) or lorazepam (1–2 mg, any route).
4. Observation for 1–2 h for signs of symptoms relief.
5. Provide a 1-d supply of benzodiazepine to be used for symptoms or on a regular basis (e.g., 4–8 doses).
6. Explanation of instructions to reliable, responsible, caring adult family member or friend.
7. Daily contact with health care provider.
8. Linkage to outpatient alcoholism treatment, primary medical care, and psychiatric care as needed.

Pharmacotherapy during the Abstinence Phase

Drug	Mechanism of Action	Dosing	Serious Adverse Effects/Contraindications
Naltrexone	Nonspecific opioid antagonist.	Titrate from 25 mg to 50 mg (average dose of 50 mg/d).	Hepatotoxicity, neuroendocrine changes. Acute opioid withdrawal, narcotic use—ensure opioid free for 14 d.
Acamprosate	Glutaminergic blockade and gamma-aminobutyric acid (GABA-A) activation.	333-mg enteric coated tablets. Titrate to effective dose over 1 week starting at half the dose to ameliorate gastrointestinal side effects. Adults >132 lb (60 kg): 2 tabs TID with meals. Adults <132 lb: 2 tabs with a.m. meal, 1 tab with midday meal, 1 tab with h.s. meal. 3 divided doses totaling 2–3 g/d.	Caution with impaired renal function.

(Continued)

---

2. Reprinted from Shader RI. *Manual of Psychiatric Therapeutics.* 3rd ed. Philadelphia: Lippincott Williams & Wilkins; 2003:149 (Table 12.5). With permission.

Drug	Mechanism of Action	Dosing	Serious Adverse Effects/Contraindications
Disulfiram	Inhibition of aldehyde dehydrogenase. Disulfiram–alcohol interaction: palpitations, flushing, nausea, vomiting, headache. In severe cases, unconsciousness, respiratory arrest, cardiovascular collapse, convulsions, and death. Have patient carry an identification card detailing the disulfiram–alcohol interaction in the event of an emergency.	Titrate as indicated from 125 mg to 500 mg p.o. qhs.	Caution with severe myocardial disease. Can exacerbate psychoses. Avoid concurrent use with metronidazole and oral hypoglycemic agents such as chlorproparmide and tolbutamide as a disulfiram-like reaction can result. Risk of hepatotoxicity, optic neuritis, peripheral neuropathy, and polyneuritis.

References

Hales RE, Yudofsky SC, *The American Psychiatric Publishing Textbook of Clinical Psychiatry*. 4th ed. Washington, DC: American Psychiatric Publishing, Inc; 2003:316–318, 347–349.

Sadock BJ, Sadock VA. *Kaplan & Sadock's Synopsis of Psychiatry: Behavioral Sciences/Clinical Psychiatry*. 9th ed. Philadelphia, Lippincott Williams & Wilkins; 2003.

Shader RI. *Manual of Psychiatric Therapeutics*. 3rd ed. Philadelphia: Lippincott Williams & Wilkins; 2003:143–167.

Chapter 40

BENZODIAZEPINE WITHDRAWAL

Guidelines for Treatment of Benzodiazepine Withdrawal[1]

1. Evaluate and treat concomitant medical and psychiatric conditions.
2. Obtain drug history and urine and blood sample for drug and ethanol assay.
3. Determine required dose of benzodiazepine or barbiturate for stabilization, guided by history, clinical presentation, drug-ethanol assay, and (in some cases) challenge dose.
4. Detoxification from supratherapeutic dosages:
   - Hospitalize if there are medical or psychiatric indications (including history of seizures and/or abuse of other drugs/alcohol), poor social supports, or polysubstance dependence or the patient is unreliable.
   - Some clinicians recommend switching to longer-acting benzodiazepine for withdrawal (e.g., diazepam, clonazepam); others recommend stabilizing on the drug that the patient was taking.
   - After stabilization reduce dosage by 30% on the second or third day and evaluate the response, keeping in mind that symptoms that occur after decreases in benzodiazepines with short elimination half-lives (e.g., lorazepam) appear sooner than with those with longer elimination half-lives (e.g., diazepam).
   - Reduce dosage further by 10% to 25% every few days if tolerated.
   - Use adjunctive medications if necessary: carbamazepine, β-adrenergic receptor antagonists, valproate, clonidine, and sedative antidepressants have been used but their efficacy in the treatment of the benzodiazepine abstinence syndrome has not been established.
5. Detoxification from therapeutic dosages:
   - Initiate 10% to 25% dose reduction and evaluate response.
   - Dose, duration of therapy, and severity of anxiety influence the rate of taper and need for adjunctive medications.
   - Most patients taking therapeutic doses have uncomplicated discontinuation.
6. Psychological interventions may assist patients in detoxification from benzodiazepines and in the long-term management of anxiety.
7. A taper over 8 to 12 weeks or longer may be indicated in patients who have been taking benzodiazepines for several years. The rate of taper can be adjusted according to patient tolerance.

---

1. Modified from Sadock BJ, Sadock VA. *Kaplan & Sadock's Synopsis of Psychiatry: Behavioral Sciences/Clinical Psychiatry*. 9th ed. Philadelphia: Lippincott Williams & Wilkins; 2003:465 (Table 12, 12-6). With permission.

Approximate Therapeutic Equivalent Doses of Benzodiazepines

Generic Name	Dose (mg)
Alprazolam	1
Chlordiazepoxide	25
Clonazepam	0.5–1
Diazepam	10
Lorazepam	2
Temazepam	20
Zolpidem	10

Adapted from Sadock BJ, Sadock VA. *Kaplan & Sadock's Synopsis of Psychiatry: Behavioral Sciences/Clinical Psychiatry.* 9th ed. Philadelphia: Lippincott Williams & Wilkins; 2003:464 (Table 12, 12-5). With permission.

Reference

Sadock BJ, Sadock VA. *Kaplan & Sadock's Synopsis of Psychiatry: Behavioral Sciences/Clinical Psychiatry.* 9th ed. Philadelphia, Lippincott Williams & Wilkins; 2003:464–465.

Chapter 41

PSYCHOTROPIC-INDUCED MOVEMENT DISORDERS

Movement Disorder	Mechanism	Onset	Clinical Features	Management
Akathisia	An imbalance between the noradrenergic and dopaminergic systems caused by the dopamine receptor antagonists.	Days to weeks	Subjective feeling of restlessness in the lower extremities, often manifested in an inability to sit still. Worsens with increasing dose.	Lower dose of antipsychotic. Switch to an atypical antipsychotic. Add propranolol 20 mg p.o. BID-TID. Benzodiazepines and clonidine are alternative treatments.
Dystonia	Dopaminergic hyperactivity in the basal ganglia that occurs when the central nervous system levels of the dopamine receptor antagonist drug begin to fall between doses.	Hours or days	Uncontrollable and painful tightening of muscles often involving spasms of neck, back, tongue, or muscles controlling lateral eye movement. Laryngeal involvement may compromise the airway and result in ventilatory difficulties. Risk factors include: young age, male gender, previous episodes of acute dystonia, recent cocaine use, hypocalcemia, and dehydration.	Acute dystonia: Diphenhydramine 25 mg IM/IV. Benztropine 2 mg IV. Follow with oral anticholinergic due to long half-lives of antipsychotics and/or continuing antipsychotic therapy. Prophylaxis: Diphenhydramine 25–50 mg p.o. BID-TID. Benztropine 1–2 mg p.o. BID. Trihexyphenidyl 5–10mg p.o. BID.
Parkinsonian syndrome	Disproportionally less dopamine than acetylcholine in the basal ganglia.	Weeks to months	Similar features of classic idiopathic Parkinson disease, such as: Diminished range of facial expression	Diphenhydramine 25–50 mg p.o. BID-TID. Benztropine 1–2 mg p.o. BID. Trihexyphenidyl 5–10 mg p.o. BID.

(Continued)

Movement Disorder	Mechanism	Onset	Clinical Features	Management
			Cogwheel rigidity Slowed movements Drooling Small handwriting Regular, coarse tremor. "Rabbit syndrome" consisting of fine, rapid movements of the lips. Can distinguish from idiopathic Parkinson disease through symmetric, bilateral signs from the onset rather than hemiparkinsonism.	Perform trial of withdrawing anticholinergic after 4–6 weeks to assess if the patient has developed a tolerance for the parkinsonian effects.
Tardive dyskinesia	Supersensitivity of postsynaptic dopamine receptors induced by long-term blockade.	Onset >6 months	Involuntary facial and oral movements, choreoathetoid movements of the extremities, and involuntary movements of the extremities and trunk. Risk factors include increasing age, duration of exposure, women, substance abuse, conventional antipsychotics. Clozapine appears to be the only agent that has not been shown to cause tardive dyskinesia.	Evaluation before treatment and every 6–12 months. No definitive treatment exists. Some studies have shown vitamin E to have some benefit, but overall data has been inconclusive.

Abnormal Involuntary Movement Scale (AIMS) Developed by the National Institute of Mental Health (NIMH)

ABNORMAL INVOLUNTARY MOVEMENT SCALE (AIMS)

(ECDEU Version)

INSTRUCTIONS: Movement Ratings: Rate highest severity observed. Rate movements that occur upon activation one *less* than those observed spontaneously.

Code: 0 = None
1 = Minimal, May be extreme normal
2 = Mild
3 = Moderate
4 = Severe

		Circle One				
FACIAL AND ORAL MOVEMENTS	1. Muscles of Facial Expression (eg. movements of forehead, eyebrows, periorbital cheeks; include frowning, blinking, smiling)	0	1	2	3	4
	2. Lips and Perioral Area (eg. puckering, pouting, and masking)	0	1	2	3	4
	3. Jaw (eg. biting, clenching, chewing, mouth opening, lateral movement)	0	1	2	3	4
	4. Tongue Rate only increase in movement both in and out of mouth, NOT inability to sustain movement	0	1	2	3	4
EXTREMITY MOVEMENTS	5. Upper (arms, wrists, hands, fingers) Include choreic movements (i.e., rapid, objectively purposeless, irregular, spontaneous). athetoid movements (i.e., slow, irregular, complex serpentine) Do NOT include tremor (i.e., repetitive, regular, rhythmic)	0	1	2	3	4
	6. Lower (legs, knees, ankles, toes) (eg. lateral knee movement, foot tapping, heel dropping, foot squirming, inversion and eversion of foot)	0	1	2	3	4
TRUNK MOVEMENTS	7. Neck, shoulders, hips (eg. rocking, twisting, squirming, pelvic gyrations	0	1	2	3	4
GLOBAL JUDGMENTS	8. Severity of abnormal movements	None, normal Minimal Mild Moderate Severe		0 1 2 3 4		
	9. Incapacitation due to abnormal movements	None, normal Minimal Mild Moderate Severe		0 1 2 3 4		

(Continued)

		No awareness	0
		Aware, no distress	1
	10. Patient's awareness of abnormal movements Rate only patient's report	Aware, mild distress	2
		Aware moderate distress	3
		Aware, severe distress	4
DENTAL STATUS	11. Current problems with teeth and/or dentures	No	0
		Yes	1
	12. Does patient usually wear dentures?	No	0
		Yes	1

References

Hales RE, Yudofsky SC. *The American Psychiatric Publishing Textbook of Clinical Psychiatry.* 4th ed. Washington, DC: American Psychiatric Publishing, Inc; 2003:1087–1091.

Kaufman D. *Clinical Neurology for Psychiatrists.* Philadelphia: W.B. Saunders Company; 2001:453.

Sadock BJ, Sadock VA. *Kaplan & Sadock's Synopsis of Psychiatry: Behavioral Sciences/Clinical Psychiatry.* 9th ed. Philadelphia, Lippincott Williams & Wilkins; 2003:1058–1061.

Sajatovic M, Ramirez LF. *Lexi-Comp's Rating Scales in Mental Health.* 2nd ed. Ohio: Lexi-Comp, Inc; 2003:228.

Chapter 42

SUBSTANCES OF ABUSE

Substance	Intoxication Signs and Symptoms	Distinguishing Characteristics of Intoxication	Urine Toxicology[a]	Withdrawal/Chronic Use
Amphetamines AKA Crank Speed	Fast onset, usually within an hour. Physical: mydriasis, anorexia, insomnia, hyperactivity—possible rhabdomyolysis, tremor, dry mouth, convulsions, chest pain, arrhythmia, heart block, coma. Psychiatric: elation, irritability, hyperactivity, depression, panic, rapid speech, psychosis.	Mydriasis Hyperactivity Psychotic symptoms	Duration of detection in urine, 48 h	Dysphoric mood, suicidality in some cases Fatigue/hypersomnia Psychomotor retardation Nightmares Chronic use: Clinical presentation similar to cocaine intoxication, but may last longer.
Cannabis AKA Marijuana Blunt Hashish Weed Pot Ganja Grass Joints Mary Jane	Physical: conjunctival injection, increased appetite, dry mouth, tachycardia, impaired motor performance, visual distortions. Psychiatric: euphoria and/or dysphoria, anxiety, paranoia, impaired judgment.	Conjunctival injection Increased appetite Dry mouth Tachycardia	Duration of detection in urine, 3 d to 4 weeks False positives: Dronabinol Naproxen	Acute withdrawal symptoms rare, but slowed cognitive processing and irritability may persist. Chronic use: Chronic use is associated with chronic obstructive pulmonary disease, lung cancer, psychiatric illness (e.g., amotivational syndrome/chronic cannabis syndrome), and cognitive dysfunction.

(Continued)

Substance	Intoxication Signs and Symptoms	Distinguishing Characteristics of Intoxication	Urine Toxicology[a]	Withdrawal/Chronic Use
Cocaine AKA Crack Coke Rock Speedballing (mixed with heroin)	Physical: mydriasis, tachycardia, elevated blood pressure, chest pain, cardiac arrhythmias, sweating or chills, gastrointestinal symptoms, anorexia, respiratory depression, dyskinesias, seizures, coma. Psychiatric: euphoria, agitation, paranoia, hallucinations, impaired judgment. Intoxication resembles mania — symptoms persisting >24–48 hrs may indicate an underlying bipolar disorder.	"Mania-like presentation" Hallucinations	Duration of detection in urine: 6–8 h Metabolites 2–4 d False positives: Fluconazole Local anesthetics	In individuals predisposed to mental illness, chronic use can lead to anxiety, panic attacks, depression, paranoia, and psychosis. Decreased fertility Early symptoms include intense drug craving, restlessness, anxiety, depression followed by fatigue, decreased energy, insomnia/hypersomnia, increased appetite. Chronic use: Chronic use may lead to apathy, persistent psychosis, cognitive impairment.
Gamma-hydroxybutyric acid (GHB) AKA Liquid ecstasy	Physical: vomiting, dizziness, respiratory depression.	Disinhibition Altered level of consciousness	Missed by routine diagnostic urine screens.	Similar to those of alcohol/benzodiazepines

Substance	Intoxication Signs and Symptoms	Distinguishing Characteristics of Intoxication	Urine Toxicology[a]	Withdrawal/Chronic Use
Grievous bodily harm "Date rape drug"	Psychiatric: euphoria, relaxed state, disinhibition. Commonly used as a recreational drug by party/night-club attendees and as a growth hormone-releaser for bodybuilders.			Anxiety and insomnia Gastrointestinal upset Tremor Feelings of doom Autonomic instability Delirium tremens-like symptoms if severe
Hallucinogens LSD (AKA Acid, Boomers, yellow sunshines) Morning glory seeds Mescaline (AKA cactus, mesc, peyote) MDA, MDEA Psilocybin (AKA magic mushroom, shrooms)	Physical: mydriasis, tachycardia, hypertension, hyperthermia. Psychiatric: mood lability, anxiety/panic, grandiosity, intensified sensations, depersonalization, derealization, hallucinations, synesthesias, hyperacusis, impaired attention/concentration, amotivation.	Visual hallucinations Synesthesias (blending of senses, e.g., sounds being seen) Intense perceptions Hyperacusis Presence of clear sensorium		No acute withdrawal syndrome. Chronic use: Psychosis Depression Flashbacks up to 30% Parkinsonian symptoms In individuals predisposed with schizophrenia, hallucinogen abuse may lead to early onset of psychosis and relapse of psychotic disorder.
Inhalants Gasoline Glue Paint thinners Spray paints	Physical: dizziness, blurred vision/diplopia, nystagmus, slurred speech, ataxia, psychomotor retardation.	"Bad trip" — syndrome of anxiety, panic, dysphoria, and paranoia. Can lead to suicidality and suicide attempts.		No acute withdrawal syndrome Chronic use: psychosis, mania, organ damage (e.g., bone marrow, kidney, liver, brain).

(Continued)

Substance	Intoxication Signs and Symptoms	Distinguishing Characteristics of Intoxication	Urine Toxicology[a]	Withdrawal/Chronic Use
AKA laughing gas, poppers, snappers, whippets	Psychiatric: belligerence, agitation, apatspaired judgment, social and occupational dysfunction.			
MDMA "Ecstasy" Adam XTC X Clarity Eve Lover's speed peace	Physical: sympathetic overload (e.g., dilated pupils, elevated heart rate and blood pressure, arrhythmias), increased tactile sensitivity, tremor, and parkinsonism. When severe, serotonin syndrome and low serum sodium. Psychological: restlessness, increased feeling of connectedness, amotivation, altered perception of time, paranoia, increased mental status, paranoia, increased libido.	Profound feeling of attachment and connectedness. Altered perception of time.		Withdrawal syndrome includes severe anhedonia, anorexia, amotivation, depressed mood. Physiological dependence uncommon. Chronic use: cognitive deficits.
Opioids Heroin (AKA brown sugar, dope, smack, H) Codeine (AKA Captain Cody, Cody) Fentanyl Morphine (AKA M, Miss Emma) Opium	Physical: miosis, slurred speech, drowsiness, staggering gait. Psychological: initial euphoria followed by depression, psychomotor retardation/agitation, impaired functioning, impaired attention and memory.	Constricted pupils Depressed mood Sedation Presence of track marks	Duration of detection in urine: Heroin 36–72 h Morphine 48–72 h Methadone 72 h False positives: Chlorpromazine	Signs and symptoms of opioid withdrawal: Physical—flu-like symptoms, nausea, abdominal cramps, vomiting, diarrhea, mydriasis, muscle and bone pain. Psychiatric—affective disorders (especially depression), anxiety, irritability.

Substance	Intoxication Signs and Symptoms	Distinguishing Characteristics of Intoxication	Urine Toxicology[a]	Withdrawal/Chronic Use
			Poppy seed Dextromethorphan Ofloxacin Rifampin	Symptomatic treatment may include NSAIDs, dicyclomine 10 mg q6h for abdominal cramps, bismuth subsalicylate 30 cc after each loose stool, and clonidine 0.1–0.2 mg p.o. q4–6h (hold for hypotension).
Phencyclidine PCP AKA Angel dust Peace pill Love boat	Physical: mydriasis, nystagmus (vertical > horizontal), hyperacusis, tachycardia, hypertension, numbness, rigidity, ataxia. Psychiatric: mood instability, aggression, altered perception, disorganization, bizarre behaviors.	Mydriasis Nystagmus (vertical > horizontal) Ataxia Diminished pain sensation Aggression	Duration of detection in urine, 8 d	Symptoms appear after several days of use and include: Depressed mood Intense drug cravings Increased appetite Bruxism Hypersomnia
Rohypnol (flunitrazepam) Commonly used as a "date rape" drug.	Physical: hypotension, dizziness, visual changes, decreased muscular tension, urinary retention. Psychiatric: decreased anxiety, loss of inhibition, altered mental status, confusion, aggression, anterograde amnesia.	Anterograde amnesia Altered mental status Decreased muscular tension		Withdrawal syndrome: Physical: headache: Tension Muscle pain Paresthesias Increased risk of seizures Photosensitivity Psychiatric: anxiety

[a]May vary widely depending upon amount ingested, compound, physical state of patient, and other factors.

References

Gahlinger PM. Club drugs: MDMA, gamma-hydroxybutyrate (GHB), Rohypnol, and ketamine. *American Family Physician.* June 2004:2619–2625.

Galanter M, Kleber HD. *The American Psychiatric Publishing Textbook of Substance Abuse Treatment.* 2nd ed. Washington, DC: American Psychiatric Publishing, Inc; 1999:151–308, 491–503, 521–529.

Hales RE, Yudofsky SC. *The American Psychiatric Publishing Textbook of Clinical Psychiatry.* 4th ed. Washington, DC: American Psychiatric Publishing, Inc; 2003:309–377.

Chapter 43

ELECTROCONVULSIVE THERAPY

General Considerations
- Uses an electrical current to depolarize the brain, inducing a generalized seizure.
- Mechanism of action unclear.
- Positive predictors include increasing age, sudden onset and short duration of illness, presence of psychotic and catatonic symptoms.
- Negative predictors include medication resistance, personality disorders.

Indications
- Typical indications include:
  - Depression, particularly delusional depression
  - Mania
  - Schizoaffective disorder, particularly mood symptoms
  - Acute psychosis in schizophrenia
  - Suicidal behavior
  - Catatonia
  - Pregnancy
  - Neuroleptic malignant syndrome
  - Obsessive compulsive disorder
  - Intractable seizures
  - Parkinson disease
- Not generally used as a first-line treatment unless rapid response to symptoms desired in conditions such as:
  - Malnutrition
  - Severe agitation, such as manic excitement
  - Elderly patients who cannot tolerate the cardiovascular, genitourinary, or central nervous system side effects of antidepressant or antipsychotic agents

Contraindications
- No absolute contraindications, including pregnancy and age limitations.
- Relative contraindications include:
  - Recent infarction, coronary artery disease, hypertension, arrhythmia
  - Conditions associated with increased intracranial pressure (e.g., intracerebral bleed/tumor)

- Conditions with increased risk for aspiration, such as gastroesophageal reflux disease
- Contraindications to anesthesia, including pulmonary conditions (e.g., chronic obstructive pulmonary disease, asthma)
- Diseases of the spinal column

Complications

- Memory deficits:
    - Acute confusional state—occurs after each treatment and is a consequence of both the seizure and the anesthetic administration. Usually lasts approximately 5 to 50 min.
    - Anterograde amnesia—impairment in the ability to recall (but not learn) information after electroconvulsive therapy (ECT). Although typically resolving within 72 h to 3 weeks, it may take 6 months to completely resolve.
    - Retrograde amnesia—memory loss for information learned before ECT. Persistent memory loss is most common for information proximal to the course of ECT, but may affect memories occurring 2 years before ECT. Although some memories initially lost may be recovered, some of the amnesia may be permanent.
    - Cognitive deficits (e.g., memory loss, confusion) may be reduced through unilateral electrode placement and the use of brief-pulse stimulation.
- Myalgia.
- Headaches, which may be pretreated with NSAIDs.
- Nausea.
- Cardiovascular complications (e.g., arrhythmias and infarction).
- Cerebrovascular complications, including intracranial bleed.
- Regurgitation and aspiration.
- Interictal ECT-induced delirium, especially in elderly patients with preexisting factors for delirium and/or medical illness (e.g., dementia, cardiovascular risk factors). Caution needed as this can result in increased risk of falls.
- Death—rare (2:100,000).

Pre-Procedure Evaluation

- Complete psychiatric, medical, neurological evaluation and physical exam focusing on risk factors
- Cognitive assessment, including evaluation of orientation and memory (anterograde and retrograde)
- Labs: complete blood cell count, CHEM 7, thyroid panel, urinalysis
- EKG
- Chest x-ray
- Appropriate medical consultation (e.g., cardiology)
- Anesthesia evaluation to determine risk of anesthesia
- Lumbosacral x-rays if spinal disease is suspected (e.g., back pain, osteoporosis)

- Neuroimaging for suspected increased intracranial pressure
- Careful documentation and detailed informed consent, preferably involving family members
- Include description of the ECT procedure, the major points of which are:
  - Pretreatment with anticholinergic drug to decrease morbidity of cardiac bradyarrthymias and aspiration
  - General anesthesia with a short-acting anesthetic and muscular relaxation with succinylcholine
  - Ventilation with 100% oxygen from the beginning of anesthesia until the patient resumes spontaneous breathing.

Pre-Electroconvulsive Therapy Checklist

- Nothing by mouth (NPO) the night before treatment.
- Ensure adequate hydration prior to NPO status.
- Careful review of all medications, only continuing medications that are absolutely necessary.
- Continue medications such as cardiac (except lidocaine), pulmonary (except theophylline, associated with status epilepticus), glaucoma (except cholinesterase inhibitors, which may prolong muscle paralysis and apneic episode), and antigastric medications.
- Avoid or decrease the doses of anticonvulsants and benzodiazepines as they raise the seizure threshold.
- Discontinue or decrease lithium doses to decrease the risk of confusion and prolonged seizures.
- Adjust the timing and doses of insulin and oral hypoglycemic agents to decrease the risk of hypoglycemia in a fasting patient.

Course of Treatment

- Acute:
  - Typical course of ECT is 6 to 12 treatments.
  - Generally given on an every-other-day basis for 2–3 weeks, usually Monday-Wednesday-Friday.
  - ECT is continued until a patient demonstrates maximal clinical response.
  - Therapy is discontinued when successive treatments do not elicit substantial improvement.
- Continuation:
  - One treatment per week for 4 weeks → then one treatment every 2 weeks for 4 weeks → then one treatment per month for 4 months.
- Maintenance:
  - ECT may be performed as an outpatient treatment every week to every several weeks.

References

Garcia KS, Lin TL, Goodenberger DM. *The Washington Manual Psychiatry Survival Guide.* Philadelphia: Lippincott Williams & Wilkins; 2003: 163–164.

Greenberg RM, Kellner CH. Electroconvulsive therapy. *Am J Geriatric Psychiatr.* 2005;13(4):268–276.

Hales RE, Yudofsky SC. *The American Psychiatric Publishing Textbook of Clinical Psychiatry.* 4th ed. Washington, DC: American Psychiatric Publishing, Inc; 2003:1122–1127.

Schatzberg AF, Nemeroff CB. *The American Psychiatric Publishing Textbook of Psychopharmacology.* 3rd ed. Washington, DC: American Psychiatric Publishing, Inc; 2004:685–707.

Chapter 44

MALINGERING

Differential Diagnosis of Malingering

DSM-IV-TR[a] Diagnosis or Condition	Intentional Production of Symptoms	Clinical Features
Conversion disorder	No	Voluntary or motor sensory deficits not explainable by a neurological or general medical condition. Typically occurs in a setting of psychological stressors.
Hypochondriasis	No	An exaggerated fear of having serious disease based on misinterpretation of benign bodily somatic symptoms. Continuing fear despite adequate medical evaluation and reassurance. Rule out delusional disorder, somatic type.
Somatization disorder	No	History of several chronic physical symptoms beginning before age 30 years that result in functional impairment. A cluster of symptoms to include 4 pain, 2 gastrointestinal, 1 sexual, and 1 pseudoneurological.
Confabulation	No	Unintentionally filling in gaps in memory with what was imagined to have happened. Often associated with disorders such as Wernicke–Korsakoff syndrome and head injury.
Factitious disorder	Yes	Voluntary production or faking of physical and/or psychological signs and symptoms. Associated with primary gain.
Malingering	Yes	Intentionally feigning, exaggerating, or lying about physical or psychological symptoms for secondary gain.

(*Continued*)

149

DSM-IV-TR[a] Diagnosis or Condition	Intentional Production of Symptoms	Clinical Features
		Secondary gain encompasses a clearly definable goal, such as housing, avoiding incarceration, financial compensation, drug seeking, medicolegal context. Often associated with antisocial personality disorder.

[a]*Diagnostic and Statistical Manual of Mental Disorders.* 4th ed. Text revision. Washington, DC: American Psychiatric Association; 2000.

Assessment

- Inconsistencies while in interview setting and otherwise.
- Inconsistencies between the patient's claimed disability and objective findings.
- Contradictions between reported previous episodes and documented psychiatric history.
- Subjective, vague, ill-defined symptoms not consistent with known clinical conditions.
- Atypical psychiatric signs and symptoms (refer to table below).
- Records or test data appear to have been tampered with.
- Collateral information including significant others, family members, friends, coworkers, employers, other involved medical providers, and law enforcement agencies.
- Review of past medical records, psychiatric records, work records, court documents, and prior disability claims.
- Psychological testing, such as the Minnesota Multiphasic Personality Inventory-2 (MMPI-2) and the Structured Inventory of Reported Symptoms (SIRS).

Clinical Features of Malingering

Signs and Symptoms	Malingering
Hallucinations	Continuous
Auditory hallucinations	Vague or inaudible Stilted language Self-report of obeying all command hallucinations
Themes	Lack a consistent theme
Association with delusions	Inconsistent

(Continued)

Signs and Symptoms	Malingering
Strategies to diminish voices	Cannot report strategies to diminish intensity of hallucinations, as opposed to the presence of developed strategies in true psychosis (e.g., listening to music, taking medications)
Visual hallucinations	Dramatic and exaggerated In black and white Miniature or giant figures
Delusions	Abrupt onset and termination Bizarre content without disordered thinking
Behavior	Eager to report their symptoms More likely to be evasive and/or intimidating

Adapted from Hales RE, Yudofsky SC. *The American Psychiatric Publishing Textbook of Clinical Psychiatry*. 4th ed. Washington, DC: American Psychiatric Publishing, Inc; 2003:701. With permission.

Management

- Malingering is a diagnosis of exclusion.
- Monitor countertransference and preserve the doctor–patient relationship.
- A nonconfrontational approach may enable the patient to give up the symptoms in response to treatment without unnecessary humiliation.
- Documentation must be written with the expectation that it will likely become a courtroom exhibit.

References

American Psychiatric Association. *Quick Reference to the Diagnostic Criteria from DSM-IV-TR*. Washington, DC: American Psychiatric Association; 2000.

Hales RE, Yudofsky SC. *The American Psychiatric Publishing Textbook of Clinical Psychiatry*. 4th ed. Washington, DC: American Psychiatric Publishing, Inc; 2003:700–702.

Resnick PJ, Knoll J. Faking it: How to detect malingered psychosis. *Curr Psychiatr*. 2005;4(11):13–25.

Sadock BJ, Sadock VA. *Kaplan & Sadock's Synopsis of Psychiatry: Behavioral Sciences/Clinical Psychiatry*. 9th ed. Philadelphia, Lippincott Williams & Wilkins; 2003:897–898.

Chapter 45

POSTPARTUM DISORDERS

	Postpartum Blues	Postpartum Depression	Postpartum Psychosis
Prevalence	50%–85%	10% of women who give birth 25% of postpartum women with history of major depression—risk further increased with intrapartum onset 50% of postpartum women with history of postpartum depression	0.1%–0.2% of all childbirths Increased risk with history of bipolar disorder, postpartum psychosis, and/or family history of mood disorders
Risk factors	History of premenstrual dysphoric disorder History of major depression Family history of depression	History of major depression Intrapartum depression Previous postpartum depression History of oral contraceptive-associated dysphoria Stressful life events Lack of support from a partner or spouse or others Unplanned pregnancy	Single Primiparous Delivery via cesarean section About 50% of deliveries associated with no perinatal complications
Course	Beginning first 2–4 d after giving birth, peaking between postpartum days 5–7 and dissipating by the end of the second postpartum week Resolves spontaneously	Onset within the first 4 weeks	Can begin within days of delivery with mean time to onset 2–3 weeks and a second peak 1–3 months after delivery Usually episodic, with subsequent episode of symptoms within a year or two after birth Subsequent pregnancies increase risk of further episodes
Clinical features	Tearfulness, mood lability, some sleep disturbance, irritability, and anxiety	Tearfulness, interpersonal hypersensitivity, sometimes mood lability, excessive anxiety, insomnia (even when the infant is sleeping and not needing attention),	Early presentation mimics postpartum blues/depression Evolves into a delirium-like, disorganized, labile, and psychotic state

(*Continued*)

	Postpartum Blues	Postpartum Depression	Postpartum Psychosis
		anhedonia, sometimes suicidal thoughts and thoughts of harming the baby, feelings of guilt and inadequacy In rare cases, severe depression may present with psychotic symptoms	Psychotic features include paranoia, delusions (e.g., defective or dead baby), and command auditory hallucinations (e.g., infanticide) Obsessive concerns about the baby's health and welfare, including feelings of wanting to harm the baby and/or themselves
Evaluation		Assessment can be aided by using the Edinburgh Postnatal Depression scale (EPDS) Thyroid function should be evaluated as the postpartum period is a time of increased risk for thyroid dysfunction.	Rule out general medical conditions, including thyroid disorders (e.g., postpartum thyroiditis, hypothyroidism), autoimmune disorders, substance use, and endocrine disorders such as Cushing and Sheehan syndrome
Treatment	No aggressive treatment required Reassurance, support, education Monitor to ensure symptoms do not persist or evolve into postpartum depression	Psychoeducation, reassurance, support Individual (cognitive, supportive, interpersonal), group psychotherapy Psychosocial assistance to decrease stressors Psychopharmacology After remission, consider continuing antidepressant medication for 6–12 months, but long term in patients with history of 3 or more episodes If there is history of postpartum depression, consider prophylactic antidepressant therapy either in the last trimester or immediately after delivery.	Considered a psychiatric emergency Acute treatment: Acute pharmacological treatment with mood stabilizers, antipsychotics, and/or benzodiazepine prn agitation Be aware of evidence available regarding safety of use during pregnancy and breastfeeding Electroconvulsive therapy should be considered for refractory postpartum psychosis

(Continued)

	Postpartum Blues	Postpartum Depression	Postpartum Psychosis
		Hospitalization Electroconvulsive therapy	Coordinate social support Pediatrician must monitor infant and get baseline behavior, sleep, and feeding patterns Indications for hospitalization include mother's fears of harming her children, obsessive concerns about the child's safety and well-being, and expressed fears of harming herself and her baby Chronic management: Monitor patient carefully when tapering medications to avoid decompensation Monitor patient for recurrence of symptoms during subsequent pregnancies and consider prophylaxis if indicated
General considerations		More likely to engage in negative parenting behaviors Older children of depressed mothers may demonstrate behavioral problems, delayed cognitive and linguistic development, and a higher risk for the development of psychiatric problems	Screening postpartum women is critical due to the estimated risk of 5% of women committing suicide and 4% committing infanticide

Resources

- Motherisk: Canadian-based program that provides information on safety or risks of drugs in pregnancy and lactation, (416) 813-6780, www.motherisk.org
- Postpartum Support International: 927 N Kellogg Avenue, Santa Barbara, CA 93111-1022, (805) 967-7636, www.postpartum.net. Provides referrals for group support, individual therapists, and psychiatrists.

- Massachusetts General Hospital Center for Women's Mental Health www.womensmentalhealth.org Web site of the Massachusetts General Hospital Reproductive Psychiatry Resource and Information Center. Provides information on pregnancy, postpartum, and psychiatric disorders.
- National Women's Health Information Center, www.4women.gov
- Depression after delivery, www.depressionafterdelivery.com
- National Institute of Mental Health, for information about Postpartum Mood Disorders, www.nimh.nih.gov

References

Friedman SH, Resnick PJ. Mothers thinking of murder: Considerations for prevention. *Psychiatric Times*. 2006; 23(10):9.

Hales RE, Yudofshy SC. *Textbook of Clinical Psychiatry*. 4th ed. Washington, DC: American Psychiatric Publishing, Inc; 2003:1519–1521.

Jacobson AM, JL. *Psychiatric Secrets*. 2nd ed. Philadelphia: Hanley & Belfus, Inc; 2001:364–367.

Sadock BJ, Sadock VA. *Kaplan and Sadock's Synopsis of Psychiatry: Behavioral Sciences/Clinical Psychiatry*. 9th ed. Philadelphia: Lippincott Williams & Wilkins; 2003:526–527.

Spinelli MG. Maternal infanticide associated with mental illness prevention and the promise of saved lives. *Am J Psychiatr*. 2004; 161(9):1548–1557.

Chapter 46

PSYCHOTROPIC MANAGEMENT IN PREGNANCY

Critical Phases in Normal Development
- Risk of termination if toxicity occurs prior to implantation.
- Prior to placenta formation, developing embryo likely not exposed to drugs.
- Weeks 3 to 8 are critical for organ development.
  - Weeks 3 to 8—cardiovascular formation.
  - Weeks 4–5 up to 16–18—neurologic development.
  - Weeks 6 to 9—lip and palate development.
- Drug exposure during later stages of pregnancy may result in decreased birth weight and poor neonatal functioning (e.g., respiratory distress).

General Principles
- Incidence of congenital malformation, 3% to 4% in the United States.
- Perform a thorough evaluation, including current mood state, maternal psychiatric history, comorbid medical disorders, obstetric history, substance use history, and prior treatment.
- Perform risk-benefit analysis to determine need for medication, keeping in mind the pregnancy period is a high-risk time for onset or relapse of psychiatric illness.
- As indicated, consider alternatives to medications, including frequent visits and psychotherapy (e.g., cognitive-behavioral).
- Factors to consider in selecting a psychotropic medication include:
  - Staying apprised of ever-changing evidence-based data on safety of use during pregnancy, including FDA risk category.
  - Preferably use agents with the most available evidence-based safety data for pregnancy/lactation. Medications with conflicting data should be avoided.
  - Of note, safety data for psychotropic use during pregnancy is limited, often conflicting, and may not be controlled for confounding factors.
  - Properties such as fewer side effects, low drug–drug interactions, low risk of hypotensive and anticholinergic effects, and few or no metabolites.
  - Consideration to potential adverse interactions with obstetric, anesthetic, and analgesic agents.

- Minimize exposure to fetus by:
  - Using the minimum dosage to achieve remission of maternal target symptoms.
  - Avoiding multiple medications.
- Monitoring
  - Continuous monitoring of maternal psychiatric target symptoms with ongoing risk-benefit analysis.
  - Documentation to support improvement of symptoms with pharmacologic treatment.
  - Consultation and coordination with obstetrician.
- Counseling and detailed informed consent including:
  - Incidence of congenital malformation 3% to 4% in the United States.
  - Risk of congenital malformation increased with psychotropic medications, particularly during weeks 6 to 10.
  - Discussion of available evidence about medication being considered, including documentation of conversation.
  - Encourage patient to involve significant other during discussion and decision making.

Antidepressants

- Selective serotonin reuptake inhibitors (SSRIs)
  - Until recently, research supported safety of SSRI use during pregnancy.
  - Recent data indicate risks of SSRI use during pregnancy, including:
    - Data on paroxetine having increased risk of major malformation, including cardiac (e.g., ventricular septal defect).
    - Studies reporting prematurity, low birth weight, serotonergic withdrawal, seizure-like activity, and poor neonatal adaptation (e.g., respiratory distress, hypoglycemia, tremulousness, altered muscle tone, jitteriness).
    - Study indicating increased risk of persistent pulmonary hypertension of the newborn (unexposed risk ~2/1000 live births).
    - One study reporting long-term effects of impairment in cognition and psychomotor skills (e.g., coordination, fine motor skills, body control).
  - Although fluoxetine has the most safety data available, its long half-life may result in neonatal complications (e.g., serotonergic withdrawal) and increased exposure to infant during breastfeeding.
  - Sertraline appears to have more favorable safety data compared to other SSRIs due to evidence indicating low transfer to fetus and favorable breastfeeding profile.
- Tricyclic antidepressants (TCAs)
  - Isolated cases of birth defects.
  - Anticholinergic effects, such as tachycardia and urinary retention.
  - Reports of withdrawal symptoms in newborns, including jitteriness, irritability, sedation, poor muscle tone.
- Important to weigh risks and benefits of antidepressant treatment given risks of untreated maternal depression (e.g., poor prenatal

care, poor nutrition, suicidality, substance use, preterm births, low birth weight, developmental delay, poor bonding with infant).

Lithium

- Birth defects:
  - 1.5 to 3 times normal incidence of birth defects.
  - 1% to 7% risk of cardiovascular malformations, including 0.1% risk of Ebstein's anomaly if used in the first trimester (10 to 20 times greater risk).
- Other risks include diabetes insipidus, premature delivery, macrosomia, goiter, floppy infant syndrome (similar to benzodiazepines), cardiac arrhythmias, hypoglycemia, polyhydramnios.
- Monitoring:
  - Obtain fetal high-resolution ultrasound and fetal echocardiogram at week 16 to 18.
  - Serial monitoring of lithium serum levels during pregnancy.
  - Prevention of dehydration and other factors that may increase lithium levels, such as NSAIDs.
  - If possible, lower lithium doses near term to avoid maternal lithium toxicity following delivery.
  - Careful monitoring of serum lithium levels after delivery due to significant fluid shifts.
- No known reports of long-term neurobehavioral effects in children.

Antiepileptic Drugs

Valproate

- Contraindicated during pregnancy.
- Dose-related neural tube defects, greatest during period of neurologic development, particularly within the first 6 weeks, when the risk is 10 to 20 times greater (including spina bifida).
- Other potential risks include:
  - Fetal valproate syndrome may include stereotypical facial features, cleft lip, cleft palate, neural tube defects, congenital heart, limb, and abdominal wall defects.
  - Withdrawal symptoms, such as irritability, altered muscle tone, seizures, vomiting, tremulousness.
  - Neurobehavioral changes, including developmental delay, cognitive impairment, and mental retardation.
- If valproate must be prescribed:
  - Avoid using during the first 6 weeks if possible.
  - Use minimum dosage necessary to target maternal symptoms.
  - Maintain maternal serum concentration <70 µg/ml.
  - Have patient take folic acid supplementation 4–5 mg/d (all women of childbearing age should take folic acid supplementation while taking valproate).
  - Prescribe oral vitamin K supplementation 10–20 mg during the last trimester of pregnancy. At birth, the newborn should receive a 1-mg injection of vitamin K.

- Monitoring:
  - Maternal monitoring, including maternal serum alpha-fetoprotein.
  - Fetal monitoring at 16 to 18 weeks gestation, including fetal echocardiogram and anatomic ultrasound.
  - Neonatal monitoring, including periodic assays of blood counts and liver function tests for nursing infants.

Carbamazepine

- Contraindicated during pregnancy.
- Dose-related neural tube defects, greatest during period of neurologic development, particularly within the first 6 weeks when the risk is 15 times greater (including spina bifida).
- Other potential risks include:
  - Fetal carbamazepine syndrome may include stereotypical facial features (e.g., up-slanting palpebral fissures, epicanthal folds, long philtrum), fingernail hypoplasia, cardiovascular abnormalities, urinary tract defects, developmental delay.
  - Theoretical toxicities, such as blood dyscrasias, coagulopathies, hepatotoxicity.
- If carbamazepine must be prescribed:
  - Avoid using during the first 6 weeks if possible.
  - Use minimum dosage necessary to target maternal symptoms.
  - Frequent serial maternal serum concentrations.
  - Have patient take folic acid supplementation 4–5 mg/d (all women of childbearing age should take folic acid supplementation while taking carbamazepine).
  - Prescribe oral vitamin K supplementation 10–20 mg during the last trimester of pregnancy. At birth, the newborn should receive a 1-mg injection of vitamin K.
  - Monitoring:
    - Maternal monitoring, including maternal serum alpha-fetoprotein.
    - Fetal monitoring at 16 to 18 weeks gestation, including fetal echocardiogram and anatomic ultrasound.
    - Neonatal monitoring, including periodic assays of blood counts and liver function tests for nursing infants.

Lamotrigine

- Limited data shows low overall rate of fetal malformations, but higher rate of miscarriages and stillbirths compared with unmedicated women.
- Possible link with cleft defects based on preliminary data collected by the North American Antiepileptic Drug (NAAED) pregnancy registry in September 2006.
- Polytherapy with valproate associated with threefold increase in major birth defects.
- Use minimum dosage necessary to target maternal symptoms.
- Frequent serial maternal serum concentrations, including pre-pregnancy baseline levels.

- Have patient take folic acid supplementation 4–5 mg/d.
- Monitoring:
  - Maternal monitoring, including maternal serum alpha-fetoprotein.
  - Monitor mother closely for evidence of toxicity after delivery due to decreased clearance of medication.
  - Fetal monitoring at 16 to 18 weeks gestation, including fetal echocardiogram and anatomic ultrasound.
  - Neonatal monitoring, including examination for drug-induced rash given immature liver function.

Antipsychotic Agents

- Little known about safety during pregnancy.
- Current evidence limited to case reports.
- High-potency agents such as haloperidol have a decreased risk for congenital malformations compared to low-potency phenothiazines.
- Olanzapine has not been shown to have an increased risk of major malformation or obstetrical complications. There is a theoretical increased risk for gestational diabetes.
- Quetiapine/risperidone—case reports of no adverse effects.
- Clozapine—case report of seizure following birth.
- Ziprasidone—no data.

Benzodiazepines

- Best to avoid during early pregnancy due to reports of increased risk of cleft lip and palate.
- Neonatal withdrawal symptoms may include lethargy, poor respiratory effort, eating difficulties, hypotonia.
- Important to weigh risks and benefits of benzodiazepine treatment given risks of untreated maternal anxiety (e.g., prolonged labor, preterm labor, fetal hypoxia).

References

Hasser C, Brizendine L, Spielvogel A. SSRI use during pregnancy: Do antidepressants' benefits outweigh the risks? *Curr Psychiatr.* 2006;5(4):31–40.

Hendrick V, Gitlin M. *Psychotropic Drugs and Women: Fast Facts.* New York: W. W. Norton & Company, Inc; 2004:54, 96–100, 124–125, 150–151.

King EZ, Stowe ZN, Newport DJ. Using antidepressants during pregnancy: An update. *Psychiatric Times,* August 2006:90–93.

Pies RP. Prenatal antidepressant use: Time for a pregnant pause? *Psychiatric Times.* September 2006:69–72.

Seeman MV. Gender differences in the prescribing of antipsychotic drugs. *Am J Psychiatr.* 2004;161(8):1328–1329.

Schatzberg AF, Nemeroff CB. *The American Psychiatric Publishing Textbook of Psychopharmacology.* 3rd ed. Arlington, VA: American Psychiatric Publishing, Inc; 2004:1118–1136.

Chapter 47

USE OF PSYCHOTROPICS IN BREASTFEEDING

General Principles

- Perform a thorough evaluation, including maternal psychiatric history.
- Perform risk-benefit analysis (of mother and infant) to determine need for medication, keeping in mind the postnatal period is a high-risk time for onset or relapse of psychiatric illness.
- Factors to consider in selecting a psychotropic medication include:
  - Data limited and often conflicting.
  - Staying apprised of evidence-based data on safety of use during breastfeeding, including FDA risk category and American Academy of Pediatrics recommendations.
  - Properties such as low milk-to-plasma ratio, short half-life, high molecular weight, high protein binding in maternal serum, relatively nonlipophilic, few or no metabolites, drug interactions, and adverse effects.
- Minimize exposure to infant by:
  - Using the minimum dosage to achieve remission of maternal target symptoms.
  - Having mother take medication immediately after breastfeeding and/or just before infant's longest sleep period.
  - Avoiding multiple medications.
  - Keeping in mind premature infants are at increased risk for adverse effects of medication due to their immature livers.
  - Supplementing with formula, which may reduce exposure to medication.
- Monitoring:
  - Continuous monitoring of maternal psychiatric target symptoms with ongoing risk-benefit analysis.
  - Documentation to support improvement of symptoms with pharmacologic treatment.
  - Consultation and coordination with infant's pediatrician.
  - Recommend monitoring of infant's well-being (e.g., feeding) and serum levels by pediatrician:
    - Lithium—serum levels, complete blood cell count (CBC).
    - Valproate/carbamazepine—liver function, CBC with platelets.

Antidepressants

- Paroxetine and sertraline appear to have low serum levels of medication exposure.
- Fluoxetine reportedly safe, but potentially greater exposure due to long half-life and case reports of neonatal colic and irritability.

- Citalopram and fluoxetine may provide greatest medication exposure.
- An 8-week double blind trial of nortriptyline and sertraline with a 16-week continuation phase demonstrated no adverse effects and low infant serum levels.
- Limited data for venlafaxine, bupropion, nefazodone, mirtazapine.

Mood Stabilizers
- Lithium
  - Generally contraindicated during breastfeeding.
  - Lethargy, hypotonia, cyanosis, and EKG changes have been reported in nursing infants.
  - An infant's immature kidney may increase risk of lithium toxicity, particularly in the setting of dehydration and fever.
  - No reports of long-term neurobehavioral sequelae.
- Carbamazepine and valproate
  - Generally considered compatible with breastfeeding.
  - Case reports of transient hepatic dysfunction (carbamazepine) and thrombocytopenia/anemia (valproate).
  - Valproate—no reports of long-term neurobehavioral sequelae.
  - Carbamazepine—case reports of adverse events, including sedation, poor suck reflex, irritability/hyperexcitability, and hepatic dysfunction.
- Lamotrigine
  - Excreted in considerable amounts in breast milk.
  - Limited data shows no adverse effects have been observed in infants, but monitor baby for life-threatening rash.
  - No reports of long-term neurobehavioral sequelae.
- Gabapentin, oxcarbazepine, topiramate
  - Insufficient data on use in breastfeeding.

Antipsychotic Agents
- Generally not recommended during breastfeeding.
- Little known about safety during breastfeeding.
- Current evidence limited to case reports.
- Small study with chlorpromazine reported no developmental deficits.
- Small study with chlorpromazine and Haldol demonstrated developmental delay.
- Olanzapine/risperidone/quetiapine—case reports without complications.
- Clozaril not recommended due to tendency to accumulate in breast milk and theoretical risk of agranulocytosis.
- Aripiprazole—unknown if excreted in breast milk.

Benzodiazepines
- Minimize use during breastfeeding.
- Case reports of sedation, poor feeding, cyanosis, and decreased respiratory rate.
- Low dose, short-acting if needed.

Further Information

- http://www.otispregnancy.org
- National Teratogen Information Services: (866) 626-OTIS
- California Teratogen Information Services: (800) 532-3749

References

Daly R. Efficacy similar for SSRIs, TCAs in postpartum depression. *Psychiatric News*. September 2006:20.

Gentile S. Clinical utilization of atypical antipsychotics in pregnancy and lactation. *Ann Psychiatr.* 2004;38:1265–1271.

Hales RE, Yudofsky SC. *The American Psychiatric Publishing Textbook of Clinical Psychiatry*. 4th ed. Washington, DC: American Psychiatric Publishing, Inc; 2003:1520–1521.

Hendrick V, Gitlin M. *Psychotropic Drugs and Women: Fast Facts*. New York: W. W. Norton & Company, Inc; 2004:59–62, 101–103, 125, 153.

Schatzberg AF, Nemeroff CB. *The American Psychiatric Publishing Textbook of Psychopharmacology*. 3rd ed. Arlington, VA: American Psychiatric Publishing, Inc; 2004:1122–1136.

Chapter 48

DRUG OVERDOSE

General Considerations

- Important to recognize overdose, but overdose is properly treated in the emergency department by a medical team.
- Because several drugs are slowly absorbed, the minimal time for observation of a suspected drug overdose should be 4 h.
- The first clinical task is to ensure the adequacy of the airway, breathing, and circulation (ABCs), which includes assessment of airway patency, respiratory rate, blood pressure, and pulse.
- Almost every overdose/loss of consciousness/coma of unknown etiology should receive IM thiamine then D5W and naloxone, which may need to be repeated.
- Caution must be used in administering neuroleptics because they can lower the seizure threshold and elicit seizures.

Distinguishing Features of Drug Overdose and Highlights of Acute Management

Medication	Toxic Dose	Signs and Symptoms	Emergency Management
Acetaminophen Due to lack of early clinical signs of toxicity, perform a Tylenol level on all patients with intentional drug OD.	7.5 g or >140 mg/kg Toxic blood levels = 15 µg/dl Rumacks Matthews nomogram—plotting acetaminophen levels vs. the time since ingestion can predict probable hepatotoxicity. Limited use in cases of chronic toxicity, time since ingestion unknown, and sustained release preparations.	7–24 h: Anorexia, nausea and vomiting, and diaphoresis. 24–48 h: Hepatic toxicity Pain in right upper quadrant with elevated liver enzymes (AST first) 72–96 h: Peak levels of hepatic enzymes and hepatic failure. Resolution phase: Symptoms abate in ~4 d; 1–3 weeks for hepatic regeneration.	Obtain baseline levels and monitor liver enzymes for at least 3 d. Activated charcoal ASAP after ingestion. *N*-acetyl cysteine (Mucomyst) 140 mg/kg p.o. as loading dose and then 70 mg/kg every 4 h until 17 doses, while continuously monitoring acetaminophen levels. Optimal use within the first 8 h. Hepatology consultation—for further management and in the event of hepatic failure to evaluate for possible liver transplant.

(Continued)

Medication	Toxic Dose	Signs and Symptoms	Emergency Management
Aspirin (acetylsalicylic acid)	Toxic → 150–300 mg/kg Lethal → 500 mg/kg Chronic ingestion = 100 mg/kg/d over several days. Toxic blood levels = 39 μg/ml Blood levels should be drawn in 6 h or more to predict further course. Draw a level 2 h until decline. Limited use in cases of chronic toxicity and sustained release preparations due to erratic and slowed absorption.	Initial symptoms include nausea, vomiting, tinnitus, hyperventilation, and altered level of consciousness. Later symptoms suggestive of a poor prognosis include lethargy, pulmonary edema, convulsions, and coma.	Stat labs for complete blood cell count (CBC), CHEM 7, arterial blood gases (ABG), and PT/PTT. Maintain continuous cardiac monitoring and pulse oximetry. Gastrointestinal (GI) decontamination with activated charcoal/ gastric lavage (within 1 h). Careful rehydration/ correction of K depletion. Alkalinize urine, monitor serum pH to prevent systemic alkalosis. Do not attempt forced diuresis. Toxic levels or any acid-base imbalance warrants an admission to an ICU and nephrology consultation.
Amphetamines	20–25 mg/kg	Mydriasis, agitation, irritability, psychotic symptoms, fever, flushing, nausea, vomiting, and diarrhea. Severe cases— rhabdomyolysis, renal failure, intracranial bleed, myocardial infarction (MI), arrhythmias, aortic dissections, seizures, coma.	Monitor CHEM 7, creatine phosphokinase (CPK), EKG. Administration of activated charcoal/ gastric lavage (for large doses). Management of agitation with benzodiazepines, avoiding neuroleptics as much as possible. Avoid restraints to prevent rhabdomyolysis. Adequate hydration to prevent acute renal failure secondary to rhabdomyolysis. Treat hyperthermia, hypertension, and arrthymias.

(Continued)

Medication	Toxic Dose	Signs and Symptoms	Emergency Management
Benzodiazepines		Drowsiness, ataxia, slurred speech, respiratory depression, coma.	Airway, breathing, and circulation. Gastric lavage/activated charcoal. Flumazenil (do not use in patients who are predisposed to or have a history of a seizure disorder)—fast action. Treat hypotension and bradycardia.
Cocaine		Initial hyperadrenergic state, with mydriasis, hypertension, tachycardia and hyperventilation, muscular twitching, agitation, altered state of consciousness. Sympathetic overload transitions into central nervous system (CNS) and cardiopulmonary depression, with complications encompassing seizures, stroke, subarachnoid hemorrhage, MI, arrhythmias, and pulmonary edema.	Baseline labs and continuous monitoring of CBC, CHEM 7, ABG, CPK, EKG. Monitor and maintain airway, breathing, and circulation. Management of agitation with benzodiazepines, avoiding neuroleptics as much as possible. Avoid restraints to prevent rhabdomyolysis. Treat rhabdomyolysis, seizures, hyperthermia, hypertension, arrhythmias, and other cardiac complications.
Phenothiazines (haloperidol, chlorpromazine, thioridazine)	150 mg/kg	Anticholinergic effects, extrapyramidal effects, cardiac complications, seizures, coma.	Airway, breathing, and circulation. Monitor CHEM 7, CPK. Continuous cardiac monitoring. Activated charcoal/gastric lavage. Emesis contraindicated. Treatment of arrhythmias, hypotension, hyperthermia, and seizures.

(*Continued*)

Medication	Toxic Dose	Signs and Symptoms	Emergency Management
Atypical antipsychotics (clozapine, olanzapine, risperidone, quetiapine, and ziprasidone)		Anticholinergic effects, CNS depression, cardiac abnormalities (hypotension, tachycardia, QT and QTc prolongation, particularly with ziprasidone). Agranulocytosis with clozapine.	Airway, breathing, and circulation. Monitor CHEM 7, CPK liver function tests (LFTs). Continous cardiac monitoring. EKG/telemetry. Activated charcoal/gastric lavage.
Tricyclic antidepressants (amitriptyline, nortriptyline, desipramine)	30–50 mg/kg lethal dose.	Erratic course, and patients may decompensate rapidly. Earliest signs—altered mental status, slurred speech, tachycardia, hypoventilation, and anticholinergic symptoms. Cardiovascular manifestations—increased QT interval, conduction defects, arrhythmias, and systemic hypotension. CNS manifestations—agitation, myoclonic jerks, seizures, and coma.	Treat hypotension, arrhythmias, and seizures. Monitor electrolytes and ABG. Serum tricyclic antidepressant levels correlate poorly with severity of toxicity. IV access, O_2 and continuous cardiac monitoring, alkalinization. Gastric lavage/multiple dose activated charcoal. Treat hypotension, arrhythmias, and seizures.
Lithium	Single ingestions of 20 mg/kg → toxic. Peak levels of $LiCO_3$ in 2–4 h post ingestion. Slow release formulations peak 6 h after ingestion. Toxicity may be secondary to dehydration, decreased dietary sodium,	**Mild intoxication** → (1.5–2.0 mEq/L) GI → Vomiting, nausea, abdominal pain, thirst. Neurological → Tremor, ataxia, dizziness, slurred speech, nystagmus, lethargy, and muscle weakness. **Moderate intoxication** (2.0–2.5 mEq/L)	Check Li levels, CHEM 7, renal function, EKG and continuous cardiac monitoring. Gastric lavage (if ingestion less then 1 h ago), emesis, sodium polystyrene sulfonate. Polyethylene glycol in the presence of rising lithium levels refractory to above treatment. Vigorous hydration and maintenance of electrolyte balance is essential.

(*Continued*)

Medication	Toxic Dose	Signs and Symptoms	Emergency Management
	and addition of thiazide diuretics, NSAIDS.	GI → persistent nausea and vomiting. Neurological → blurred vision, muscle fasciculations, myoclonus, hyperactive deep tendon reflexes, choreoathetoid movements, convulsions, delirium, coma, hemodynamic failure. **Severe intoxication** → Lithium level >2.5 mEq/L Seizures, cardiac arrhythmias, coarse tremors, hypotension, renal failure, and death.	Hemodialysis indicated for Li level >4.0 mEq/L, renal failure, altered mental status, seizures, arrhythmias, and pulmonary edema. Continue checking lithium levels until two consecutive levels show a downward trend.
Phencyclidine		Agitation, hallucinations, hypertension, hyperpyrexia, tachycardia, vertical nystagmus, rhabdomyolysis, decreased sensitivity to pain. Stupor, coma, analgesia, seizures, respiratory depression, renal failure secondary to rhabdomyolysis.	Monitor electrolytes, CPK and BUN/Cr. Supportive treatment. Management of agitation with benzodiazepines, avoiding neuroleptics as much as possible. Minimize stimulation and caution due to increased risk of violence. Restraints should be avoided due to risk of rhabdomyolysis. Decontamination measures such as gastric lavage may be countertherapeutic by way of increasing agitation.
Selective serotonin reuptake inhibitors (fluoxetine, sertraline, paroxetine, citalopram)		Altered mental status, confusion, vertigo, ataxia, psychosis, GI symptoms (nausea and vomiting), tachycardia, rare	Monitor EKG (especially with citalopram) and for any symptoms that are suggestive of serotonin syndrome. Gastric lavage/activated charcoal.

(Continued)

Medication	Toxic Dose	Signs and Symptoms	Emergency Management
		arrhythmias and seizures.	Treat arrhythmias, seizures.
Valproate		Somnolence, confusion, GI upset progressing to respiratory depression, arrhythmias, pancreatitis, and drug-induced hepatitis and coma.	Check CHEM 7, LFTs, amylase, lipase, CBC with differential. Continuous cardiac monitoring. Supportive management including respiratory support, gastric lavage. Treat seizures.

This table presents characteristic features of drug overdose and general principles of acute management. Please refer to a detailed clinical reference for comprehensive management.

References

Galanter M, Kleber HD. *The American Psychiatric Publishing Textbook of Substance Abuse Treatment.* 2nd ed. Washington DC: American Psychiatric Publishing, Inc; 1999:151–308, 491–503, 521–529.

Green GB, Harris IS, Lin GA, et al., eds. *The Washington Manual of Medical Therapeutics.* 31st ed. Philadelphia: Lippincott Williams & Wilkins; 2004:565–590.

Hales RE, Yudofsky SC. *The American Psychiatric Publishing Textbook of Clinical Psychiatry.* 4th ed. Washington, DC: American Psychiatric Publishing, Inc; 2003:309–377.

Chapter 49

DRUG-INDUCED NEUROLOGICAL SYNDROMES

Characteristic	Neuroleptic Malignant Syndrome (NMS)	Central Anticholinergic Syndrome	Serotonin Syndrome	Malignant/ Lethal Catatonia	Malignant Hyperthermia
Risk factors	Rapid increases and high doses of antipsychotic medication IM antipsychotic use Dehydration/poor nutrition, comorbid medical illness Young age Male Presence of mood disorder Previous episode of NMS	Elderly	Concurrent use of ≥ 2 serotonergic agents (e.g., selective serotonin reuptake inhibitors [SSRIs], monoamine oxidase inhibitors [MAOIs], L-tryptophan, meperidine, lithium) High doses (dose-related)	Young adults (mean age = 33 years) Women Schizophrenia, manic or depressed mood states Comorbid infection, metabolic, other medical conditions	Genetic predisposition Neuromuscular disorder (e.g., myopathy)
Typical symptoms	Altered mental status Lead-pipe rigidity Autonomic instability Hyperthermia	Decreased: Salivation/sight/sweat Lacrimation Urination Bowel movements	Gastrointestinal symptoms (diarrhea, nausea/emesis)	Extreme hyperactivity ("catatonic excitement") and progressive hyperthermia before onset of stupor	Hyperthermia with muscular rigidity s/p recent administration of an anesthetic agent
Clinical features	Altered mental status Hyperthermia Confusion/agitation Rigidity/tremor Autonomic instability (hypo- or hypertension, tachycardia, high fever, diaphoresis	Altered mental status Fever Dilated, sluggish pupils/blurred Change in mental status/delirium Flushed skin	Altered mental status Diaphoresis Flushing/sweating Shivering/restlessness Tremor Akathisia	Altered mental status Fever Confusion Violent and self-destructive behavior (e.g., no p.o. intake) Mood lability	Hyperthermia Muscular rigidity Arrhythmias Ischemia Diaphoresis Hot skin Mottled cyanosis

(*Continued*)

Characteristic	Neuroleptic Malignant Syndrome (NMS)	Central Anticholinergic Syndrome	Serotonin Syndrome	Malignant/Lethal Catatonia	Malignant Hyperthermia
	Extrapyramidal symptoms (dystonia, akinesia, tremor, cogwheeling, lead-pipe rigidity)	Dry skin and mucous membranes Dry mouth Urinary retention Constipation/absent bowel sounds Hallucinations Tachycardia	Myoclonus High fever Elevated blood pressure Hyperreflexia Ataxia Rhabdomyolysis	Rigidity/waxy flexibility Psychotic symptoms Autonomic instability: tachycardia, diaphoresis, elevated or labile blood pressure	Hypotension Rhabdomyolysis
Mechanism	Sudden decrease in central dopaminergic function after blockade of dopamine receptors at multiple sites (e.g., basal ganglia, hypothalamus)	Excessive blockade of acetylcholine receptors	Overactivation of central 5-HT receptors	Reduced dopaminergic functioning within the basal ganglia-thalamo-cortical circuits	Inherited disorder triggered by a halogenated inhaled anesthetic (e.g., Halothane) and/or depolarizing muscle relaxant (e.g., succinylcholine), causing increased calcium levels in skeletal muscle.
Lab findings	Elevated creatine phosphokinase (CPK) (>300 U/mL) Elevated white blood cell count (>10 K/mm³) Increased aldolase, alkaline phosphatase, AST, ALT Low serum Fe, Ca, and Mg Hypo/hypernatremia Myoglobinuria	No specific lab findings	Acute renal failure	Elevated CPK Leukocytosis Transaminitis Decreased serum Fe	Elevated CPK Acute renal failure Disseminated intravascular coagulation Respiratory/metabolic acidosis Hyperkalemia Hypermagnesemia

Characteristic	Neuroleptic Malignant Syndrome (NMS)	Central Anticholinergic Syndrome	Serotonin Syndrome	Malignant/ Lethal Catatonia	Malignant Hyperthermia
Management	Thorough medical/neurological and mental status evaluation and exam Discontinue all medications Supportive measures (cooling, hydration, nutrition, aspiration precautions, anticoagulation) Consider dopaminergic agonist (bromocriptine 5 mg BID-TID), dantrolene and/or electroconvulsive therapy (ECT) may help While restarting the neuroleptic: Consider reintroduction of antipsychotic no earlier than 2 weeks after resolution of NMS Use lowest effective dosage of antipsychotic agent, but monitor closely for relapse	Discontinue suspected agent Acute reversal may entail IV physostigmine 1–2 mg (1 mg/min) but do not use for maintenance treatment (risk of bradycardia, nausea/emesis, seizures) Supportive measures (cooling, hydration)	Discontinue suspected agent(s) Supportive measures (e.g., cooling, hydration, respiratory, pain management, nutrition) Additional agents—dantrolene, bromocriptine, propanolol, methysergide, and cyproheptadine (serotonin antagonist) may be helpful Mechanical ventilation	Hold antipsychotic drugs Rule out comorbid medical illness Watch for medical complications Supportive measures (e.g., hydration, maintenance of nutritional status) Benzodiazepines (e.g., lorazepam 1–2 mg p.o./IM BID-TID) ECT if above ineffective	Dantrolene 100% O_2 Supportive measures (e.g., cooling, $NaHCO_3$, hydration)
Mortality	Mortality ~20%			Mortality ~9%	Mortality rare (most commonly with medication combinations containing MAOIs)

References

Bernstein CA, Ladds BJ, Maloney AS. *On Call Psychiatry*. Singapore: W.B. Saunders Company; 1998:130–132.

Caroff SN, Mann SC, Francis A, et al., eds. *Catatonia: From Psychopathology to Neurobiology*. Arlington, VA: American Psychiatric Publishing, Inc; 2004:107–115.

Hales RE, Yudofshy SC. *Textbook of Clinical Psychiatry*. 4th ed. Washington, DC: American Psychiatric Publishing, Inc; 2003:1059, 1091–1092.

Northoff G. Catatonia and neuroleptic malignant syndrome: Psychopathology and pathophysiology. *J Neural Transmission*. 2002; 109:1453–1467.

Richard IH. Acute, drug-induced, life-threatening neurological syndromes. *Neurologist*. 1998;4(4):196–208.

Rundell JR, Wise MG. *Consultation Psychiatry*. 3rd ed. Washington, DC: American Psychiatric Publishing, Inc; 2000:180–190.

Sadock BJ, Sadock VA. *Kaplan and Sadock's Synopsis of Psychiatry: Behavioral Sciences/Clinical Psychiatry*. 9th ed. Philadelphia: Lippincott Williams & Wilkins; 2003: 993–994, 998, 1059, 1066.

Schatzberg AF, Nemeroff CB. *The American Psychiatric Publishing Textbook of Psychopharmacology*. 3rd ed. Arlington, VA: American Psychiatric Publishing, Inc; 2004:239, 437–438, 524, 557.

Chapter 50

PHYSICAL HEALTH MONITORING FOR PSYCHOTROPIC MEDICATIONS

Mood Stabilizers

Lithium

Test	Baseline	Weekly for 4 Weeks	Monthly for 3 Months	Quarterly	Yearly	When Symptoms Arise	Special Considerations
Pregnancy test	X					X	In women of childbearing age. Category D. 0.1–0.7% absolute risk of Ebstein's anomaly of tricuspid valve (normal population = 0.01%).
Complete blood count	X					X	Most frequently benign leukocytosis >15 K white blood cell count (WBC)/mm^3. Reverses with discontinuation. Exclude infection.
Blood chemistries (including renal tests)	X				X	X	Discontinue if fluctuating or unstable renal function and consult with medicine/nephrology.
ECG	X				X	X	Indicated in patients >40 years and/or history of cardiac disease. Discontinue with sinus disease or conduction defects. May reveal transient T wave inversion/flattening that often normalizes with either continuation or discontinuation of lithium.
Urinalysis	X					X	Management of lithium-induced nephrogenic diabetes insipidus (often reversible if lithium discontinued). 1. Increase fluid intake. 2. Consider K 10–20 mEq/d.

Test	Baseline	Weekly for 4 Weeks	Monthly for 3 Months	Quarterly	Yearly	When Symptoms Arise	Special Considerations
							3. Consider thiazide (caution), amiloride (non-thiazide & preferred) 5–10 mg p.o. BID.
							4. Discontinue lithium.
							5. Continue electrolyte monitoring. If lithium must be continued, decrease to lowest effective dose & QD if able. Monitor lithium level minimum q 2 months. Proteinuria indicative of glomerular & tubule damage.
Thyroid function tests	X				X		Increased risk in women & rapid cyclers. Usually reversible hypothyroidism. Evaluate for signs/symptoms and refer to endocrinology. May continue if adequately treated & monitored.
Serum plasma concentrations	X	X	X	X		X	0.8–1.2 (lower in elderly). Toxicity possible at lower serum concentrations. Monitor for clinical symptoms of toxicity.
Weight/body mass index (BMI)/waist circumference					X		Possible mechanism due to polydipsia, carbohydrate & lipid metabolism, glucose tolerance. Diet, exercise & low-calorie liquids.

Adapted from Gelenberg AJ. Laboratory and other testing for patients taking psychotropic medications. *Biological Therapies in Psychiatry* 2004;27(11):41-44.

Hyperparathyroidism—If you observe back pain, kyphoscoliosis, osteoporosis, hypertension, cardiomegaly, impaired renal function in a patient with elevated calcium, check PTH levels and consult endocrinology.

Valproic Acid

Test	Baseline	2 Weeks	Monthly for 6 Months	Quarterly	Every 6 Months	Yearly	When Symptoms Arise	Special Considerations
Pregnancy test	X						X	In women of childbearing age. Neural tube defects 1%–2% first trimester.
Complete blood count with platelets and differential	X		X		X		X	Clinically significant thrombocytopenia rare.
Blood chemistries	X		X		X		X	At high doses, mild to moderate hyponatremia due to syndrome of inappropriate antidiuretic hormone secretion (SIADH). Reversible when lower dose)
Serum plasma concentrations				X			X	50–125 mcg/ml trough levels.
Prothrombin time	X				X		X	Monitor liver function.
Weight/BMI/ waist circumference	X					X		Common. Not dose dependent.

(Continued)

Test	Baseline	2 Weeks	Monthly for 6 Months	Quarterly	Every 6 Months	Yearly	When Symptoms Arise	Special Considerations
Amylase							X	Rare cases of pancreatitis. Most commonly first 6 months.
Liver function	X						X	Liver function tests optional. Discontinue if >2.5 times normal AST/ALT. Plasma NH$_3$ often increased transiently and may not necessarily mandate interruption of treatment.
Serum androgen assays							X	Symptoms of polycystic ovarian syndrome include obesity, hirsutism, amenorrhea.

Adapted from Gelenberg AJ. Laboratory and other testing for patients taking psychotropic medications. *Biological Therapies in Psychiatry*. 2004;27(11):41–44.

Carbamazepine

Test	Baseline	2 Weeks	Monthly	Quarterly	Annually	When Symptoms Arise	Special Considerations
Pregnancy test	X					X	In women of childbearing age. Increased risk of spina bifida, microcephaly, craniofacial defects, finger nail hypoplasia. Potent inducer of hepatic enzymes. May cause failure of oral contraceptives. Recommend barrier contraception as well.
Complete blood count	X	X	X	X		X	Monthly for 3 months. Rapid-onset agranulocytosis & aplastic anemia 1/125 K. Immediate management of sore throat, fever, rash, petechiae, bruising. Discontinue if WBC <3000/mm³, absolute neutrophil count (ANC) <1500/mm³, platelets (PLT) <100 K/mm³.
Liver function tests	X	X	X	X		X	Monthly for 3 months. Discontinue if ALT/AST >3 times upper limit of normal.
Blood chemistries	X				X	X	SIADH with secondary hyponatremia. Check electrolytes with weakness, altered mental status, headache. Refer to hyponatremia section in Chapter 10 for management.
Thyroid function test	X				X		May reduce T3, T4, TSH. Rarely clinically significant but should refer to endocrinology.
Serum plasma concentrations		X		X		X	4–12 mcg/mL.

Adapted from Gelenberg AJ. Laboratory and other testing for patients taking psychotropic medications. *Biological Therapies in Psychiatry*. 2004;27(11):41–44.

Second-Generation Antipsychotics (SGA)

Test	Baseline	4 Weeks	8 Wks	12 Wks	Quarterly	Yearly	Special Considerations
Pregnancy test	X						In women of childbearing age. Category C.
Personal/family medical history	X					X	Assess for risk of metabolic syndrome, dyslipidemia, coronary artery disease, hypertension, diabetes, obesity.
Weight/BMI	X	X	X	X	X		Caution in using in patients with BMI ≥ 25. Unless BMI ≤18.5 (underweight), an increase of 1 BMI unit or waist circumference >40 in. for men and >35 in. for women, & >5% weight gain of initial weight requires intervention (nutrition, physical activity counseling, program referral with expertise in weight management) and may include switching SGA.
Waist circumference	X					X	Measure at level of umbilicus. Males with a waist circumference >40 in. and women >35 in. and two risk factors for cardiovascular disease are at increased risk for diabetes mellitus and coronary artery disease, regardless of BMI.
Blood pressure	X			X		X	Measure orthostatic hypotension in elderly. If BP >140/90 mm Hg (130/80 in diabetic patients), ensure appropriate treatment initiated. Refer to appropriate health professional.
Fasting plasma glucose	X			X		X	More frequent monitoring needed for diabetic and overweight/obese patients. Watch for symptoms of new-onset diabetes.

Test	Baseline	4 Weeks	8 Wks	12 Wks	Quarterly	Yearly	Special Considerations
Fasting lipid profile	X			X		X	Refer to Chapter 18. Refer to primary care provider if LDL >130 mg/dl. Reduce fat intake.
QT interval prolongation		X	X				Antipsychotics with increased risk for QTc prolongation include thioridazine, mesoridazine, ziprasidone, pimozide. Baseline EKG indicated with heart disease, history of syncope, family history of sudden death at early age, congenital prolonged QT syndrome.
Prolactin and sexual function	X*	X		X		X	Mainly for antipsychotics associated with prolactin elevation (e.g., thioridazine, risperidone). During the first few weeks, ask women about sexual function, breast changes (galactorrhea), and menstruation. In men inquire about erectile/ejaculatory disturbances and hypogonadism. Increased risk of osteoporosis and breast and endometrial cancer. Monitor for premature menopause symptoms. If signs/symptoms continue and/or prolactin level still elevated, refer to endocrinology.
Extrapyramidal symptoms and tardive dyskinesia	X	Weekly first 2 weeks & after dose increase			For high-risk & elderly, q3 months for first	q6 months for first generation and yearly for second generation	Refer to Abnormal Involuntary Movements scale (AIMS) in Chapter 41.

(Continued)

Test	Baseline	4 Weeks	8 Wks	12 Wks	Quarterly	Yearly	Special Considerations
					generation and q6 months for second generation		
Cataracts						Yearly inquiry. q6 months slit-lamp for Seroquel. Yearly evaluations for patients >40 years and q2 years for young patients.	Inquire about vision change, especially distance vision and blurry vision. Ensure routine ocular evaluations (q5years for Seroquel). Pigmentary retinopathy associated with thioridazine.

Copyright © 2004 American Diabetes Association. From *Diabetes Care*, Vol. 27, 2004;596–601. Reprinted with permission from The American Diabetes Association. Marder SR, Essock SM, Miller AL, et al. Physical health monitoring of patients with schizophrenia. *Am J Psychiatr*, 2004;161 (8):1334–1349.

Clozaril

In addition to the tests listed in the table on the next page, orthostatic blood pressure should be measured weekly until the dose is stable and then monthly in the elderly. Do not initiate in patients with history of myeloproliferative disorder or clozapine—induced agranulocytosis or granulocytopenia.

Test	Baseline	Weekly for 6 Months	Every Other Week from 6 Months	Once or Twice per Year	Inadequate Response or Adverse Effects	Special Considerations
Weight/BMI	X	X	X			Body weight increases by 10% or more in many patients. Provide nutritional counseling at initiation of treatment. Weight gain may not plateau until year 4 and may not be dose related.
Waist circumference	X			X		See recommendations under SGA above.
White blood cell count and neutrophil count	X	X	X	After 12 months or 4 weeks		1. Initial WBC count must be $\geq 3500/mm^3$ and ANC $\geq 2000/mm^3$. 2. If WBC count is $2000-3000/mm^3$ or the ANC is $1000-1500/mm^3$, interrupt tx and monitor for signs of infection. Check CBC with differential daily until WBC $>3000/mm^3$ and ANC $>1500/mm^3$, then twice-weekly. If no symptoms of infection, and WBC returns to $>3500/mm^3$ and ANC $>2000/mm^3$, can rechallenge with clozapine and monitor weekly for 1 year. 3. If WBC $<2000/mm^3$, or the ANC $<1000/mm^3$, discontinue tx and do not rechallenge pt. Monitor until normal and for at least 4 weeks from day of discontinuation, treat infection, coordinate care with medicine.

Test	Baseline	Weekly for 6 Months	Every Other Week from 6 Months	Once or Twice per Year	Inadequate Response or Adverse Effects	Special Considerations
Fasting glucose	X					New-onset diabetes mellitus can occur at rate of about 7%/year & not necessarily associated with weight gain. See SGA recommendations above.
Orthostatic blood pressure measurement		X				Weekly until dose is stable then monthly in elderly.
Serum troponin level						Check WBC count if myocarditis suspected. Warrants urgent referral to medicine.
Fasting lipid panels	X			X		See SGA recommendations above.
Serum plasma concentrations					X	Serum level >350 ng/ml may be associated with higher response rate. Check in nonresponders. Duration of treatment to assess response is 3–6 months.

Adapted from Gelenberg AJ. Laboratory and other testing for patients taking psychotropic medications. *Biological Therapies in Psychiatry.* 2004;27(11):41–44.

References

Gelenberg AJ. Laboratory and other testing for patients taking psychotropic medications. *Biological Therapies in Psychiatry.* 2004;27(11):41–44.

Goff DC, "Medical morbidity and mortality in schizophrenia: Guidelines for psychiatrists. *J Clin Psychiatr.* 2005;66(2):183–192.

Hales RE, Yudofsky SC. *American Psychiatric Publishing Textbook of Clinical Psychiatry.* 4th ed. Washington, DC: American Psychiatric Publishing, Inc; 2003:1104–1113.

Marder SR, Essock SM, Miller AL, et al. Physical health monitoring of patients with schizophrenia. *Am J Psychiatr.* 2004; 161(8):1334–1349.

Sadock B, Sadock V. *Kaplan & Sadock's Pocket Handbook of Psychiatric Drug Treatment.* 3rd ed. Philadelphia, Lippincott Williams & Wilkins; 2001:87–95, 136–147, 252–258.

Chapter 51

SUICIDE ASSESSMENT AND MANAGEMENT

Suicide Risk Factors

Demographic	Findings on History	Examination Findings	Protective
Male gender White Single/not married Age Homosexual/bisexual orientation Unemployed	**History of present illness** Presence of suicidal behavior, suicidality, and/or efforts made to avoid intervention Presence of ambivalence/regret for surviving suicide attempt Termination gestures (e.g., updated will, suicide note) Identified precipitating events Reluctant to accept help Difficulty coping Access to weapons **Past psychiatric history** Presence of mental illness History of personality disorders Previous suicide attempts Poor treatment compliance **Substance history** Comorbid substance abuse **Past medical history** Comorbid medical illness/pain Terminal illness **Family history** Family history of suicide **Social history** History of abuse Positive beliefs about death (as per religion) Poor social support	Severe anxiety Agitation/restlessness Altered mental status Impulsivity Pervasive insomnia Intense affective state or apathy Impaired concentration Rumination Hopelessness/lack of future orientation Psychotic symptoms	Responsibilities including to family, children, pets, and/or work Life satisfaction Religion Past evidence of demonstrating strong coping skills and problem solving Presence of therapeutic alliance with providers Compliance with treatment plan

General Principles of Management

- Inpatient hospitalization is warranted for high-risk patients.
- A treatment plan should include the following:
  - Management of psychiatric symptoms, particularly anxiety/agitation and insomnia.
  - Treat substance abuse.
  - Consider close observation/24-h supervision as indicated.
  - Remove lethal means and document discussion with patient and significant others.
  - Coordinate treatment plan with family and/or significant others.
  - Exploration of social support to decrease social isolation and to provide for safety and empathy.
  - Frequent visits for serial suicide risk assessments, including careful documentation.
  - "No harm" contracts:
    - Do not protect against malpractice liability.
    - Patient refusal to sign may indicate increased risk.
    - Should include a crisis plan in the event of suicidality (e.g., calling 911 and/or designated support person).
- Electroconvulsive therapy may be indicated for severe and/or refractory depression, psychotic depression, and/or catatonic features.
- Chronic suicidal ideation:
  - Acute suicide risk can coexist with chronic suicidal ideation/suicidal gestures.
  - Monitor your countertransference reactions during suicide risk assessments.
- Risk management considerations should include the following:
  - Documentation
    - Suicide risk assessment.
    - Discussions with patient/significant others/other providers involved in patient's care.
    - Treatment plan including rationale for current treatment, any changes made, and crisis/safety plan.
    - Consultation(s)/second opinions.
  - Actions
    - Removal of firearms.
    - Frequent visits for serial suicide risk assessments.
    - Careful pharmacologic management to avoid risk of overdose with limited supply.
    - Frequent communication with significant others.
    - Maintenance of therapeutic alliance with patient.
  - After a completed suicide attempt
    - Notify malpractice insurance carrier.
    - Consultation with risk management.
    - Communication with patient's family while maintaining patient confidentiality and documentation of conversation.

Resources

24-hour nationwide hotline access 1-800-SUICIDE (1-800-784-2433)
http://www.suicidehotlines.com

References

Jacobs DG. *Practice Guideline for the Assessment and Treatment of Patients with Suicidal Behaviors.* Arlington, VA: American Psychiatric Association; 2004:835–907.

Mays D. Structured assessment methods may improve suicide prevention: Standard patient interview processes can mislead clinicians about acute risk factors. *Psychiatr Ann.* 2004;34(5):367–372.

Shader RI. *Manual of Psychiatric Therapeutics.* 3rd ed. Philadelphia: Lippincott Williams & Wilkins; 2003:229–239.

Chapter 52

HERBALS AND DIETARY SUPPLEMENTS

General Considerations

- Herbal agents are considered food supplements, and safety, optimal dosing, and efficacy do not have to be established.
- As herbal agents are not subject to U.S. Food and Drug Administration (FDA) regulations, there may be variations in potency and possibility of contamination.
- Significant drug-drug interactions may occur with psychotropic medications.
- There is limited evidence-based safety data for use during pregnancy and lactation.

Common Psychoactive Herbs and Food Supplements

Name	Use	Adverse Effects	Interactions	Comments
Black cohosh	Menopausal: hot flashes and mood symptoms Premenstrual dysphoric disorder	Weight gain, gastrointestinal (GI) upset, headache, dizziness. Possible life-threatening liver toxicity. Monitor liver function.	Hepatotoxic herbs/supplements/drugs: may increase liver toxicity. Hormone-sensitive cancers and conditions: limited data, should avoid use. Breast cancer: limited data suggesting increased risk for metastasis.	Most studies used doses of 40–80 mg BID, but doses may vary.
DHEA (dehydroepiandrosterone)	Depression Menopausal symptoms Schizophrenia Anti-aging	Masculinization Liver disease Possible exacerbation of metabolic syndrome, including insulin resistance.	Cytochrome P450 3A4 substrates: may increase levels due to enzyme inhibition. Hormone-sensitive cancers and conditions, including breast and prostate cancers; limited data suggesting increased risk. Converted into androgens and estrogens and may have adverse effects on pregnancy and nursing infants.	Doses range from 25–100 mg/d.
Ephedra	*Banned by FDA due to cardiovascular and cerebrovascular events.* Weight loss agent Used as a recreational drug "herbal ecstasy"	Serious adverse effects may include hyperadrenergic state (e.g., arrhythmias, tachycardia, hyperthermia), exacerbation of narrow angle glaucoma, psychosis, mania, suicidality, cardiac arrest, seizures, stroke, death.	Synergistic with sympathomimetics, serotonergic agents. Avoid with monoamine oxidase inhibitors (MAOIs). QTc prolongation: increased risk of serious ventricular arrhythmias. Decreased effectiveness of anticonvulsants and antidiabetics.	May cause false-positive urine amphetamine or methamphetamine test results.

(Continued)

Name	Use	Adverse Effects	Interactions	Comments
Ginkgo	Cognitive/memory impairment Depression Premenstrual dysphoric disorder Schizophrenia Antidepressant-induced sexual dysfunction	Allergic skin reactions, GI upset, dizziness, muscle spasms, headache, possible induction of mania, lowered seizure threshold.	Anticoagulants/antiplatelet drugs: concomitant use may increase risk of bleeding. Anticonvulsants: reduced effectiveness. Cytochrome P450 1A2/2D6 substrates: mild inhibitor. Cytochrome P450 2C19: inducer. Cytochrome P450 2C9: strong inhibitor. Trazodone: concomitant use associated with coma.	Doses range from 120–240 mg/d. Prevailing mechanisms of action are through antioxidants, free radical scavenging properties, improvement of circulation. Studies report improved cognition in dementia of Alzheimer's type.
Ginseng	Stress reduction agent Stimulant for chronic fatigue Depression Immune system booster	Ginseng abuse syndrome with insomnia, hypertonia, and edema. Induction of mania.	Antidiabetes drugs: increased glucose-lowering effects with resultant hypoglycemia. Decreased effectiveness of antipsychotic drugs, MAOIs, warfarin. Potentiation of activity of stimulants. Women with hormone-sensitive conditions (e.g., breast, uterine, ovarian): limited data, avoid use.	Doses range from 1–3 g/d. Teratogenic effects in animal models: avoid use during pregnancy. Limited data for use in breast feeding.
Kava Kava	*Associated with life-threatening hepatic damage.* Sedative/hypnotic	Increased risk of suicide with comorbid depression. GI upset, headache, dizziness, lethargy, sedation, unsteady gait, anticholinergic,	Potentiation of activity of anxiolytics, alcohol. Decreased effectiveness of dopamine agonists.	Dose ranges from 60–240 mg of active ingredient daily.

Name	Use	Adverse Effects	Interactions	Comments
	Anxiolytic Antispasmodic	extrapyramidal symptoms, impaired cognition. DO NOT USE before driving or operating heavy machinery.		
Melatonin	Insomnia Circadian-based sleep disorders Benzodiazepine withdrawal	Uncommon, but high doses may worsen depression and cause abdominal cramps, fatigue, headache, dizziness. Very high doses can exacerbate depression.	May interact with antihypertensive agents.	Dose ranges from 0.3–10 mg/d.
Omega-3 fatty acids Fish oils - EPA, DHA Plant-derived-ALA	Triglyceride-lowering agent Coronary artery disease; anti-inflammatory, antithrombotic Bipolar disorder/depression Dementia of Alzheimer's type	GI side effects, including fishy aftertaste, halitosis, nausea, diarrhea. Sedation. Induction of mania.	Anticoagulant/ antiplatelets: increased risk of bleed. Potentiation of antihypertensive drugs. Implantable defibrillators: increased risk of ventricular arrhythmias.	Dose ranges from 3000–9000 mg/d. Fatty/fish oils may contain significant amounts of toxins (e.g., mercury, PCBs) that can be carcinogenic, teratogenic, immunosuppressive, or lead to central nervous system (CNS) disturbances.
SAMe	Depression Fibromyalgia	GI upset, dry mouth, headache, sweating, dizziness.	Additive serotonergic/ MAOI effects with increased risk of serotonin syndrome.	Dose ranges from 400–2400 mg/d.

(Continued)

Name	Use	Adverse Effects	Interactions	Comments
St. John's wort	Depression Anxiety Somatization disorder	Anxiety. Induction of mania. Activation, GI upset, dizziness, headache, neuropathy, insomnia, photodermatitis, photosensitivity, withdrawal syndrome. Induction of mania, psychosis. Contraindicated in pregnancy, lactation, cardiovascular disease, and pheochromocytoma.	Levodopa: reduced effectiveness. Oral contraceptives: increased/abnormal intermenstrual, menstrual bleeding. Non-nucleoside reverse transcriptase inhibitors(NNRTIs) and protease inhibitors: decreased serum levels. Cytochrome P450 1A2/ 2C9/3A3/3A4: inducer.	Doses range from 300–1800 mg/d. Stop using at least 3 d before starting an agent with serotonergic properties. Limited data regarding teratogenic effects: avoid use during pregnancy. Avoid use during breastfeeding due to reports of colic and lethargy.
Valerian	Anxiety Insomnia Benzodiazepine withdrawal	Headache, GI upset, activation, daytime sedation, drowsiness with resultant cognitive impairment. Cardiac dysfunction and hepatotoxicity with long-term use. Hepatotoxicity. DO NOT USE before driving or operating heavy machinery.	Avoid concomitant use with alcohol, benzodiazepines, CNS depressants due to additive therapeutic and adverse effects. Cytochrome P450 CYP 3A4: inhibitor.	Doses range from 400–900 mg of valerian extract daily.

Name	Use	Adverse Effects	Interactions	Comments
Vitamin E Alpha-tocopherol	Dementia of Alzheimer's type	Uncommon but can cause GI upset, fatigue, headache, blurred vision, rash.	Anticoagulant/antiplatelet potential, particularly in combination with warfarin and/or antagonism of vitamin K-dependent clotting factors: increased risk of bleeding. Cytochrome P450 3A4: inducer.	Dose ranges from 400–2000 IU daily.
	Other dementias such as vascular, mixed, Huntington's Premenstrual dysphoric disorder Tardive dyskinesia			Retrospective data indicating concurrent use with Aricept may help slow cognitive decline in dementia of Alzheimer's type. Therapeutic effects attributed to antioxidant properties.

Some data included in this table are derived from single case reports and anecdotal evidence; solid clinical evidence is lacking, doses may vary depending upon formulation and are intended to be a guideline.

References

Beaubrun G, Gray GE. A review of herbal medicines for psychiatric disorders. *Psychiatric Services.* September 2000:1130–1134.

Edie CF, Dewan N. Which psychotropics interact with four common supplements. *Curr Psychiatr.* 2005; 4(1):17–29.

Kaplan BJ, Kaplan VA. *Kaplan and Sadock's Pocket Handbook of Psychiatric Treatment.* 3rd ed. Philadelphia: Lippincott Williams & Wilkins; 2001:289–294.

Natural Medicines Comprehensive Database. www.naturaldatabase.com (last updated October 18, 2005).

Schatzberg AF, Cole JO, DeBattista C. *Manual of Clinical Psychopharmacology.* 4th ed. Arlington, VA: American Psychiatric Publishing, Inc; 2003:595–611.

Section V

Appendices

Appendix 1

INITIAL PSYCHIATRIC EVALUATION

1. Identifying data
   - Name
   - Age
   - Sex
   - Language best understood/spoken
   - Ethnicity/race
   - Marital status
   - Reliability/source of current information
2. Chief compliant: "___"
3. History of present illness
   - Details of current hospitalization, including details of the events that brought the patient in
   - Psychiatric review of systems: depressive/manic/psychotic/anxiety/eating disorder symptoms
4. Past psychiatric history
   - Age of onset of psychiatric symptoms
   - Course of psychiatric symptoms
   - History of past hospitalizations
   - History of past suicide attempts, including the details of past attempts
   - History of outpatient follow-up with medication history
   - History of violence
5. Medication history
   - Medication trials
   - Response to medications taken in the past, including both positive and negative effects
   - History of compliance with medications
   - History of electroconvulsive therapy or other somatic treatments
6. Past medical/surgical history, including medical review of symptoms
   - Particularly history of head trauma with/without loss of consciousness
   - History of hepatitis B/HIV (especially in patients with history of IV drug use)
   - History of seizure disorder
7. Allergies
8. Family history of psychiatric illness, including suicide, substance use, mental retardation, and neurological history
9. Substance abuse history
   - History of current use, including substances used, amount, route of use, and withdrawal symptoms

- History of when first used, patterns of past use
- History of past/current substance abuse treatment
- History of risk-taking behaviors, including sharing needles

10. Social history
    - Where born and raised, including the patient's recollection of what his or her childhood was like
    - History of abuse in childhood: physical/sexual/emotional/verbal abuse
    - Education history
    - Occupational history
    - Relatedness to others: marriages, children, family ties, and social support
    - Financial support and housing
    - Religious history, including beliefs about life after death in a suicidal patient
    - Legal history

Appendix 2

MENTAL STATUS EXAM

General Appearance
- Approximate age and comparison to stated age, sex, habitus, grooming and hygiene, clothing, distinguishing features.

Behavior
- Carriage and mannerisms, reaction and attention to environment, range of motoric activity, eye contact.
- Useful adjectives: rigid, distractible, psychomotor agitation/retardation, fixed gaze, fleeting.

Interpersonal Manner
- Demeanor, attitude, interaction with interviewer.
- Useful adjectives: guarded, restrained, suspicious, glib, seductive, entitled, preoccupied.

Speech
- Rate, rhythm/cadence, volume, spontaneity, level of description, articulation, prosody/tone.
- Useful adjectives: pressured, stammering, verbose, slurred, monotone, irritable prosody.

Mood
- Prevailing and underlying emotion.
- Useful adjectives: dysphoric, elevated, euphoric, angry, anxious.

Affect
- Facial expressions, temporal component, modulation, appropriateness, range.
- Useful adjectives: blunted, flat, restricted, labile, stable, full, wide, shallow.

Thought Process
- Manner in which ideas are linked, flow of patient's thoughts, fluency.
- Useful adjectives: linear, goal-oriented, circumstantial, tangential, loosening of associations, blocking, neologisms, clanging.

Thought Content
- Nominal themes and subtext, hallucinations, delusions, illusions, suicidal ideation, homicidal ideation.

Insight
- Understanding and implications of current issues.

Judgment
- Decision-making and problem-solving abilities.

Cognitive Functioning
- May include testing for orientation, attention, concentration, memory, general knowledge, abstraction (similarities, differences, proverb interpretation).

Appendix 3

NEUROLOGIC EXAM

Mental Status

Please refer to Appendix 2.

Cranial Nerves

- I (olfactory): smell
- II (optic): visual acuity/fields, funduscopic exam
- III, IV, VI (oculomotor, trochlear, abducens): eyelid opening, pupil sizes and reactivity, extraocular movements
- V (trigeminal): corneal reflex, facial sensation, strength of muscles of mastication
- VII (facial): strength of upper and lower facial muscles, anterior two thirds taste (tongue)
- VIII (vestibulocochlear): hearing
- IX-X (glossopharyngeal, vagus): articulation, palate movement, swallowing, gag reflex, posterior taste (tongue)
- XI (spinal accessory): sternocleidomastoid and trapezius muscles (lateral head movement, neck flexion, shoulder shrug)
- XII (hypoglossal): tongue movement/strength (protrusion from mouth, lateral)

Sensation

- Light touch, pain, temperature, vibratory
- Joint position

Motor

- Extremity muscle strength
- Abnormalities such as rigidity, spasticity, flaccidity, fasciculations, akinesia/bradykinesia
- Presence of involuntary movements, including tremor, chorea, tics, dystonia, myoclonus

Reflexes

- Deep tendon reflexes: biceps, triceps, brachioradialis, quadriceps, patellar, ankle jerk, plantar
- Abnormal reflexes, including babinski sign (upgoing toes)

Cerebellar

- Finger-to-nose
- Heel-to-shin
- Rapid alternating movements

Equilibrium

- Romberg
- Test for drift (e.g., look for pronator drift)
- Gait exam, including tandem, walking on toes/heels

Higher Cortical Function

- Mental status, including orientation, concentration, language and speech, memory, praxis
- Simultaneous double stimulation
- Primitive reflexes, including glabellar, snout, suck/root, grasp, palmomental, perseveration
- Presence of neglect
- Stereognosia and graphesthesia

References

Kaufman DM. *Clinical Neurology for Psychiatrists*. Philadelphia: W.B. Saunders Company; 2001:3–7.

Lindsay KW, Bone I. *Neurology and Neurosurgery Illustrated*. London: Churchill Livingstone; 1999:4–28.

Maxwell RW. *Maxwell Quick Medical Reference*. 3rd ed. Tulsa, Oklahoma Maxwell Publishing Company, Inc; 1996.

Willms JL, Schneiderman H, Algranati PS. *Physical Diagnosis: Bedside Evaluation of Diagnosis and Function*. Baltimore: Williams & Wilkins; 1994:472–500.

Appendix 4

NEUROPSYCHOLOGICAL TESTING

Psychological Testing

- Psychological testing encompasses areas that include intellectual ability, academic achievement, adaptive behavior, and personality characteristics.
- Commonly performed tests include:
  - Wechsler Intelligence scales, which measure general intellectual ability, including general fund of knowledge and vocabulary.
  - Minnesota Multiphasic Personality Inventory, a measure of psychological functioning, abnormal behavior.
  - Bender Visual Motor Gestalt test.
  - Rorschach Inkblot test for personality styles and characteristics.
  - Sentence completion tests.
  - Thematic Apperception test for self-concept, relations to others, including motivations, emotions, core personality conflicts.
  - Millon Clinical Multiaxial inventories, for identification of Axis I and personality disorders.

Neuropsychological Testing

- Neuropsychological testing, which includes measures of sensory perceptual functions, motor functions, psychomotor problem solving, language and communication skills, executive function, and other cognitive skills and abilities.
- May help diagnose brain damage and/or brain dysfunction, assist with rehabilitation planning, and elicit cognitive strengths and weaknesses.
- Commonly performed tests include:
  - Luria-Nebraska Neuropsychological Battery
  - Halstead Reitan Neuropsychological Battery
  - Wisconsin Card Sorting test

References

Hales RE, Yudofsky SC. *Textbook of Clinical Psychiatry.* 4th ed. Washington, DC: American Psychiatric Publishing, Inc; 2003:190–211.

Spar JE, Rue AL. *Concise Guide to Geriatric Psychiatry.* 3rd ed. Washington, DC: American Psychiatric Publishing, Inc; 2002:163–165.

Stern TA, Herman JB. *Massachusetts General Hospital Psychiatry Update and Board Preparation.* New York: McGraw-Hill; 2004:239–247.

INDEX

A

Abdominal pain, 2–3
Abnormal involuntary movement scale, 136–137
Acamprosate, 130
Acarbose, 20
Acetaminophen overdose, 164
Acetylcholinesterase inhibitors, 93–94
Actos. *See* Pioglitazone
Acute abdomen, 3
Acute confusional state, 146
Acute pancreatitis, 14
Acyclovir, 115
Aggression, 108–110
Agitation, 121–122
AIDS. *See* HIV/AIDS
Akathisia, 134
Alcohol intoxication and withdrawal, 127–131
Alpha-adrenergic blockers, 47
Alpha-glucosidase inhibitors, 20
Alpha-tocopherol, 198–199
Alprazolam, 133
Alzheimer's dementia, 89–90
Amantadine, 109
Amaryl. *See* Glimepiride
Ambien. *See* Zolpidem
Amitriptyline, 106, 167
Amlodipine, 47
Amphetamines, 139, 165
Amphotericin B, 115
Anaphylaxis, 4–5
Angiotensin II receptor blockers, 47
Angiotensin-converting enzyme inhibitors, 47
Anterior cerebral artery, 78
Anterograde amnesia, 146
Anticonvulsants, 94
Antidepressants
 during breastfeeding, 161–162
 for dementia, 94
 during pregnancy, 157–158
 for sleep disorders, 106
Antidiabetic agents, 20–21
Antiemetics, 56
Antiepileptic drugs, 158–160
Antihistamines, 4
Antipsychotics
 during breastfeeding, 162
 for chronic aggression, 110
 for dementia, 94
 health monitoring during use of, 183–186
 overdose of, 166–167
 during pregnancy, 160
 for sleep disorders, 106
Anxiety, 102, 114
Anxiolytics, 94
Aortic dissection, 11
Arrhythmias, 7–8
Aspirin overdose, 165
Atazanavir, 115
Atenolol, 47, 129
Atrioventricular block, 7–8
Avandia. *See* Rosiglitazone
Azithromycin, 63

B

Basilar artery, 78
Benazepril, 47
Benzodiazepines. *See also specific drug*
 during breastfeeding, 162
 overdose of, 166
 during pregnancy, 160
 for sleep disorders, 105
 withdrawal from, 132–133
Benztropine, 134

Beta-blockers, 47, 110
Beta-lactam antibiotics, 115
Biguanides, 20
Bilirubin, 61
Bisacodyl, 17
Bite, human, 43
Black cohosh, 195
Blood alcohol level, 127
Bradyarrhythmias, 7–8
Bradykinesia, 99
Breastfeeding, 161–163
Bright light therapy, 105
Bromocriptine, 109
Bundle branch blocks, 7
Bupropion SR, 59

C

Calcium-channel blockers, 47
Cannabis, 139–140
Capacity, 125–126
Carbamazepine
  during breastfeeding, 162
  health monitoring during use of, 181–182
  during pregnancy, 159
  for seizures, 110
Casts, in urine, 62
Cataracts, 186
Catatonia, 171–173
Cefixime, 63
Ceftriaxone, 63
Cellulitis, 9
Central anticholinergic syndrome, 171–173
Centrally acting adrenergic agents, 47
Cephalexin, 9
Chest pain, 10–15
Chlordiazepoxide, 133
Chlorpromazine, 123, 166
Ciprofloxacin
  for cystitis, 63
  for prostatitis, 63
  for pyelonephritis, 64
Citalopram, 109, 161, 168
Citrucel. *See* Methylcellulose
Clonazepam, 133
Clonidine, 47
Clozapine, 100, 160, 167
Clozaril, 187–189
Cocaine, 140, 166
Codeine, 142–143
Cognitive decline, 91–92
Cognitive impairment, 86
Colace. *See* Docusate sodium
Confabulation, 149
Constipation, 16–18
Contraception, emergency, 35
Conversion disorder, 149
Cortical dementia, 88
Co-trimoxazole, 115
Crystals, in urine, 62
Cycloserine, 115
Cystitis, 63

D

Dalmane. *See* Flurazepam
Dehydration, 86
Dehydroepiandrosterone. *See* DHEA
Delavirdine, 115
Delirium
  characteristics of, 83–87
  in HIV, 113–114
  traumatic brain injury and, 108
Dementia
  of the Alzheimer type, 89–90
  cortical, 88
  differential diagnosis, 83
  epidemiology of, 88
  frontotemporal, 89–90
  HIV-associated, 113
  with Lewy bodies, 91
  management of, 93–95
  outpatient management, 95
  post-stroke, 91
  resources about, 95–96
  safety considerations, 95
  stages of, 92–93
  subcortical, 88
  vascular, 90–91
  work-up for, 92
Depression
  differential diagnosis, 83
  in HIV patients, 114
  postpartum, 152
  sleep disorders and, 102
  after traumatic brain injury, 109

Desipramine, 167
Dextroamphetamine, 109
DHEA, 195
DiaBeta. *See* Glyburide
Diabetes mellitus, 19–22
Diabetic ketoacidosis, 21–22
Diazepam, 76, 133
Dicloxacillin, 9
Didanosine, 115
Dietary supplements, 194–200
Diphenhydramine
  for anaphylaxis, 4
  for dystonia, 134
  for sleep disorders, 106
Disulfiram, 131
Diuretics, 47
Docusate sodium, 17
Donepezil, 93, 109
Doxycycline, 63
Drug overdose, 164–169
Drug-induced neurological syndromes, 171–173
Dulcolax. *See* Bisacodyl
Dyspepsia, 23–26
Dyspnea, 27–28
Dystonia, 134

E
Efavirenz, 115
Electrocardiogram, 6–8
Electroconvulsive therapy, 145–148
Electrolyte disturbances, 29–34
Emergency contraception, 35
Ephedra, 195
Epigastric pain, 2
Epinephrine, 4
Epithelial cells, in urine, 61–62
Eszopiclone, 105
Ethinyl estradiol, 35

F
Factitious disorder, 149
Falls, 36–37
Fentanyl, 142–143
Fever, 38–39
Fish oils, 197
Fluoxetine, 109, 161, 168–169
Flurazepam, 105

Fosamprenavir, 116
Foscarnet, 116
Frontotemporal dementia, 89–90

G
Gabapentin, 162
Galantamine, 94
Gamma-hydroxybutyric acid, 140–141
Gastritis, 13
Gastroesophageal reflux disease, 24–25
Ginkgo, 196
Ginseng, 196
Glimepiride, 20
Glipizide, 20
Glucophage. *See* Metformin hydrochloride
Glucotrol. *See* Glipizide
Glucotrol XL. *See* Glipizide
Glyburide, 20
Glynase. *See* Glyburide
Glyset. *See* Miglitol

H
H_2 blockers, 24
Halcion. *See* Triazolam
Hallucinations, 150–151
Hallucinogens, 141
Haloperidol
  for agitation, 123
  for delirium, 84–85
  overdose of, 166
Headache, 69–70
Hepatitis A, 40
Hepatitis B, 40
Hepatitis C, 40–42
Hepatitis D, 41
Hepatitis E, 41
Herbal agents, 194–200
Heroin, 142–143
HIV/AIDS
  counseling about, 111–112
  medications for, 115–116
  neuropsychiatric assessment, 112–115
Human bite, 43
Huntington disease, 97–98
Hydralazine, 47

Hydrochlorothiazide, 47
Hyperglycemic hyperosmolar state, 21–22
Hyperkalemia, 32–33
Hypernatremia, 29–30
Hypertension
  classification of, 45
  description of, 44
  lifestyle modifications for, 46
  pharmacologic treatment of, 46–47
Hypertensive emergency, 48
Hypertensive urgency, 48–49
Hyperthyroidism, 50–51
Hypochondriasis, 149
Hypogastric pain, 3
Hypokalemia, 33–34
Hypomania, 102
Hyponatremia, 30–32
Hypothyroidism, 50–51

I

Inhalants, 141
Insomnia, 103–106
Insulin, 21
Interferon, 41–42, 58
Interferon-α, 116
Internal carotid artery, 78
Intracranial hemorrhage, 71–72
Isoniazid, 116

K

Kava kava, 196–197
Ketones, 61

L

Lactulose, 17
Lamivudine, 116
Lamotrigine
  during breastfeeding, 162
  for mania, 109
  during pregnancy, 159–160
Lansoprazole, 25
Laxatives, 17
Left bundle branch block, 7
Left lower quadrant pain, 2
Left upper quadrant pain, 2
Left ventricular hypertrophy, 7

Levonorgestrel, 35
Lisinopril, 47
Lithium
  during breastfeeding, 162
  health monitoring during use of, 175–178
  overdose of, 167–168
  during pregnancy, 158
Lorazepam
  for agitation, 123
  for alcohol withdrawal, 129
  dosing of, 133
  for seizure disorder, 76
Lunesta. *See* Eszopiclone

M

Magnesium hydroxide, 17
Malignant hyperthermia, 171–173
Malignant/lethal catatonia, 171–173
Malingering, 149–151
Mania, 102, 114
MDMA, 142
Melatonin, 197
Memantine, 94
Mental status examination, 203–204
Metabolic syndrome, 52–53
Metamucil. *See* Psyllium
Metformin hydrochloride, 20
Methotrexate, 116
Methylcellulose, 17
Methylphenidate, 94, 109
Metoprolol, 47
Micronase. *See* Glyburide
Middle cerebral artery, 78
Miglitol, 20
Mild cognitive impairment, 93
Mild neurocognitive disorder, 113
Millon Clinical Multiaxial inventories, 206
Mini-Mental State Exam, 84
Minnesota Multiphasic Personality Inventory, 206
Mobitz type I block, 8
Mobitz type II block, 8
Morphine, 142–143
Movement disorders, psychotropic-induced, 134–137

Multiple sclerosis, 73–74
Myocardial ischemia, 11

N

Naltrexone, 130
Nateglinide, 20
Nausea and vomiting, 54–56
Neuroleptic malignant syndrome, 171–173
Neurologic examination, 205–206
Neuropsychological testing, 206
Nicotine gum, 60
Nicotine inhaler, 59–60
Nicotine lozenges, 60
Nicotine nasal spray, 59
Nicotine patch, 59
Nifedipine, 47
N-methyl-*D*-aspartic acid antagonists, 94
Nonepileptiform seizure disorder, 76
Nortriptyline, 167

O

Ofloxacin
  for cystitis, 63
  for prostatitis, 63
  for pyelonephritis, 64
Olanzapine
  for aggression, 109
  for agitation, 123
  for delirium, 85
  overdose of, 167
Omega-3 fatty acids, 197
Omeprazole, 25
Opioids, 142–143
Opium, 142–143
Osmotic laxatives, 17
Overdose, 164–169
Oxcarbazepine, 162

P

P wave, 6
Pain
  abdominal, 2–3
  chest, 10–15
Pancreatitis, acute, 14
Pantoprazole, 25

Parkinson disease, 99–101
Parkinsonian syndrome, 134–135
Paroxetine, 161, 168
Pentamidine, 116
Peptic ulcer disease, 13, 25
Pericardial tamponade, 12
Pericarditis, 12
Periumbilical pain, 2
Phencyclidine, 143, 168
Phenothiazines, 166
Pioglitazone, 20
Pneumothorax, 13
Postconcussion syndrome, 108
Posterior cerebral artery, 78
Postpartum blues, 152
Postpartum depression, 152
Postpartum psychosis, 152
Posttraumatic epilepsy, 108
PR interval, 6
Prandin. *See* Repaglinide
Prazosin, 47
Precose. *See* Acarbose
Pregnancy, 156–160
Prevacid. *See* Lansoprazole
Prilosec. *See* Omeprazole
Procarbazine, 116
Propranolol, 110, 129
Prostatitis, 63
Protease inhibitors, 112–113
Proteinuria, 61
Proton pump inhibitors, 24
Protonix. *See* Pantoprazole
Psilocybin, 141
Psychiatric evaluation, 201–202
Psychosis
  in HIV/AIDS, 115
  postpartum, 152
Psychostimulants, 94
Psychotropics. *See also specific drug*
  during breastfeeding, 161–163
  movement disorders induced by, 134–137
  during pregnancy, 156–160
Psyllium, 17
Pulmonary embolism, 12
Purified protein derivative, 57
Pyelonephritis, 64

Q

Q waves, 6
QRS complex, 6
QRS interval, 6
QT interval, 6, 8
QTc prolongation, 8
Quetiapine
  for aggression, 109
  for delirium, 85
  overdose of, 167
  for Parkinson disease, 100
  during pregnancy, 160
  for sleep disorders, 106
Quinolones, 116

R

R wave, 7
Ramelteon, 105–106
Ranitidine
  for anaphylaxis, 4
  for gastroesophageal reflux disease, 24
Red blood cell count, 61
Relaxation therapy, 104
Repaglinide, 20
Restoril. *See* Temazepam
Restraint, 122
Retrograde amnesia, 146
Ribavirin, 42
Right bundle branch block, 7
Right lower quadrant pain, 3
Right upper quadrant pain, 2
Right ventricular hypertrophy, 7
Risperidone
  for delirium, 85
  overdose of, 167
  during pregnancy, 160
  for psychosis, 109
Rivastigmine, 93–94
Rohypnol, 143
Rorschach Inkblot test, 206
Rosiglitazone, 20
Rozerem. *See* Ramelteon

S

SAMe, 197
Schizophrenia, 83, 102
Seclusion, 122
Seizure disorder, 75–77
Selective serotonin reuptake inhibitors. *See also specific drug*
  during breastfeeding, 161
  for dementia, 94
  overdose of, 168–169
  during pregnancy, 157
Senna, 17
Serotonin syndrome, 171–173
Sertraline, 109, 168
Shortness of breath, 27–28
Sinus rhythm, 6
Sleep disorders, 102–106
Sleep hygiene, 104
Sleep restriction therapy, 105
Smoking cessation, 59–60
Somatization disorder, 149
Sonata. *See* Zaleplon
St. John's wort, 198
ST segment, 7
Starlix. *See* Nateglinide
Status epilepticus, 76
Stavudine, 116
Stimulant laxatives, 17
Stimulus control therapy, 104–105
Stool surfactants, 17
Stroke
  characteristics of, 79–80
  dementia after, 91
  localization of, 78
Subcortical dementia, 88
Substance abuse, 102, 114, 139–144
Suicide
  assessment of, 191
  HIV/AIDS, 114–115
  management principles, 192–193
  risk factors for, 191
  traumatic brain injury and, 108
Sulfonamides, 116
Sulfonylureas, 20

T

T wave, 7
Tachyarrhythmias, 7
Tarasoff v. University of California Regents, 124
Tardive dyskinesia, 135, 185–186

Tegaserod, 17
Temazepam, 105, 133
Tension pneumothorax, 13
Thematic Apperception test, 206
Thiabendazole, 116
Thiazolidinediones, 20
Thyroid disorders, 50–51
Topiramate, 162
Transient ischemic attack, 79–80
Traumatic brain injury, 107–110
Trazodone, 106, 110
Triazolam, 105
Tricyclic antidepressants, 157, 167
Trihexyphenidyl, 134
Trimethoprim/sulfamethoxazole
   for cystitis, 63
   for prostatitis, 63
   for pyelonephritis, 64
Tuberculosis screening, 57–58

U
Urethritis, 63
Urinalysis, 61–62
Urinary tract infections, 63–64
Urine pH, 61

V
Valerian, 198
Valproate
   for agitation, 123
   during breastfeeding, 162
   overdose of, 169
   during pregnancy, 158–159
Valproic acid, 109–110, 178–180
Valsartan, 47
Vascular dementia, 90–91
Vasodilators, 47
Ventricular hypertrophy, 7
Vertebral artery, 78
Vinblastine, 116
Vincristine, 116
Violence, 121–124
Viral hepatitis, 40–42
Vitamin E, 198–199
Vomiting. *See* Nausea and vomiting

W
Wechsler Intelligence scales, 206
Wenckebach block, 8
White blood cell count, 61
Withdrawal
   from alcohol, 127–131
   from benzodiazepines, 132–133

Z
Zalcitabine, 116
Zaleplon, 105
Zantac. *See* Ranitidine
Zelnorm. *See* Tegaserod
Zidovudine, 116
Ziprasidone, 123, 160, 167
Zolpidem, 105, 133
Zyban. *See* Bupropion SR